Matthias Gerschwitz

Beyond the Virus

HIV infected my blood but not my life

I0494420

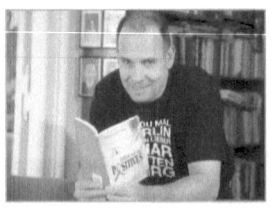 Matthias Gerschwitz, born 1959, the youngest of six children, was raised in Solingen, a German town between Cologne and Düsseldorf. After his university graduation, he moved to Frankfurt and for seven years worked as product and promotion manager for a mid-sized manufacturer of household products. Subsequently, he went to work for an international fragrance and flavor company near Cologne. He has lived in Berlin since 1992 where he has been working as a marketing consultant. He started publishing books in 2007, initially focusing on his fondness for history. His books explore the history of old brands, renowned landmarks, long-established companies or institutions like old bars, houses or stores.

In »Beyond the Virus«, Gerschwitz combines personal experience and relevant information about the immune disease HIV, with which he got infected in the early 90s.

MATTHIAS GERSCHWITZ

BEYOND THE VIRUS

HIV INFECTED MY BLOOD BUT NOT MY LIFE

IMPRINT

»Beyond the Virus«	© 2015 by Matthias Gerschwitz
Based on:	Matthias Gerschwitz: »Endlich mal was Positives« (part 1: 2009 / part 2: 2015) published by BoD, Norderstedt/Germany
Translation:	Vivian Romney & Matthias Gerschwitz
Corrections:	Michael Madison
Cover Photo:	Jan Dettmer
Website:	http://www.beyond-the-virus.com
Contact:	btv@gerschwitz.com
Imprint of record:	CreateSpace Independant Publishing Platform / CreateSpace-assigned ISBN
Printed by:	On-Demand Publishing LLC 100 Enterprse Way, Suite A200 Scotts Valley, CA 95066 – U.S.A. www.createspace.com
ISBN-13:	978-1518857973
ISBN-10:	1518857973

To
Vivian

I am glad we have been close friends
for more than thirty years.

Matthias Gerschwitz is gay, and he is HIV positive. The virus was detected in 1994, but likely transmitted in 1992. In 2009, he wrote a book about his life with the virus in German titled: »Endlich mal was Positives«, which translates to: *Finally, Something Positive (to report)*. The author is one of more than 80,000 HIV infected persons in Germany (as of October 2015) and one of the only a few to go public with his infection. The tone of the book corresponds with his personal way to handle his infected life: pro-actively, openly and with optimism. In 2009, Gerschwitz was named »Ambassador of World AIDS Day« for Germany. In 2010, his book was honored with the »Annemarie Madison Award«, a German award named after an early Californian AIDS activist. Also in 2010, he starred in a video »Living together positively – and safe« for the German government's official AIDS education campaign. In November 2014, The Deutsche Welle, Germany's international TV broadcaster, produced a video for German, English, Spanish and Arab speaking countries about the author, his book and his infection.

In February 2015, Gerschwitz published a sequel to »Endlich mal was Positives« dealing with the current social and health care situation of people infected with HIV in Germany. The book documents that HIV positive people are still subject to discrimination and criminalization.

»Beyond the Virus« covers the author's personal circumstances, experiences and insights. Some general information also found its way into »Beyond the Virus«, thus connecting the personal insight with interesting and relevant knowledge on how HIV is viewed in Germany today.

TABLE OF CONTENTS

About this book   9

Preface   11

Getting started   13

Going back in history   15

Another closet to come out of   21

Positive in the (German) gay community   35

How did it happen?   39

On my way to treatment   41

A positive attitude is a good start   47

The daily dose   51

Good news about the treatment   55

In the long run we're all dead   61

Fate or guilt?   63

Dream a little dream of … protection   66

It has nothing to do with me   69

Lust for life   75

beyond-the-virus.com

»There are worse things in life than death.
Have you ever spent an evening with an
insurance salesman?«
(Woody Allen)

ABOUT THIS BOOK

When people talk about HIV today, some call it a disease; some don't. And yet others think of it as just an infection. Those who are infected or dealing with it emphasize modern antiretroviral drugs that enable them to lead almost normal lives. Those not touched by HIV still emphasize the danger of infection and the fatal course of the disease.

But do people really talk about HIV?

No. Those who are infected are afraid to speak because they fear isolation, discrimination and even criminalization. So many reports prove these fears are justified. Others not affected by HIV do not want to hear or talk about something they do not want to be contaminated by.

In 2012, more than thirty years after the first cases in California, an official survey in Germany about HIV and AIDS came out. The results showed that 45% of the interviewees felt they were not thoroughly informed about the immune deficiency disease, although the *German Federal Center for Health Education* has been active for over twenty-five years with their campaign »Gib AIDS keine Chance« (*Don't give AIDS a chance*). Cuts in financial subsidies for the work of self-help groups in the 90s left only reduced scope for badly needed means of prevention.

But cuts cannot be the only reason for the information deficit from the survey. Indeed, although funding has declined since the mid-90s, other organizations, like local

AIDS self-help groups and health authorities, activists and even a handful of infected persons have continued to spread the word about HIV reality. There are many sources of information about the disease, but the will to use them seems to be lacking. Still too many people think HIV is restricted to the so-called risk groups, such as homosexuals and drug addicts. And in addition, they ignore the medical progress of the last twenty years. And still too many people refer to HIV as AIDS, although there is a great difference: being HIV positive does not necessarily mean to suffer from AIDS.

HIV can strike anyone; the virus is not picky. It does not care if you are male or female, or hetero-, bi- or homosexual. But HIV is one of the very few incurable diseases from which one can protect oneself. To ensure that, unbiased knowledge is necessary. This book is meant to impart exactly that.

PREFACE

»Beyond The Virus« is about life with HIV, now spanning over more than twenty years. Matthias Gerschwitz, author and protagonist, never bemoaned his diagnosis. Instead he accepted the infection rather quickly and proceeded to deal with his altered life with optimism and a positive attitude. Andreas Schultz, a high school classmate, remembers the birth of the original German »Endlich mal was Positives« book in 2009:

»I only found out that Matthias Gerschwitz was infected with HIV by coincidence. In 2003, while compiling the invitation list for the 25th anniversary of our high school graduation, a former classmate volunteered the information: ›Matthias has AIDS, didn't you know?‹ Although nobody had spread the word, there was only one thought: ›Is he still alive?‹ We sent him an invitation anyway.

In those days my image of HIV was very simple. We all had seen the movie ›Philadelphia‹ with Tom Hanks and knew that HIV meant AIDS and AIDS meant DEATH. So I was very happy to see Matthias at the reunion and even happier to find him safe, sound and full of life. Since then, we have become close friends.

Matthias had contemplated writing a book about his life with HIV for some time. He only needed an additional push to put thought into action. While lingering in a Berlin bar on a warm summer evening, I encouraged him to write about his experiences. I was sure his thoughts would be helpful and educational for many people. I thought the time was ripe for such a book and he seemed ready to tackle the challenge. Only a few days later I received the first thirty pages, a couple of weeks later the work was completed.

The result is a book that delivers insight into an infection. It is written for those who want to know more about HIV regardless if they have the infection themselves and, of course, for those who have to cope with the infection of a family member or a friend. Here someone is talking about his HIV infection who has never forgot to live and laugh.

Matthias's story inspires hope, but not a false sense of security. Today HIV and AIDS have waned from public awareness, although the number of new infections in developed countries has not decreased. So HIV prevention still is of critical importance. This book provides education in a friendly, quiet, and charming way without admonishing or moralizing. Moral philosophy will not help the adolescent who is infected at his first hetero- or homosexual encounter. Nor will it help the allegedly irreproachable citizen, who after an extramarital escapade suddenly finds himself part of a fringe group suffering from what sometimes still is called ›gay plague‹.

This book confronts the reader with unpopular facts. But closing one's eyes to the facts would not change them for the better anyway. More input is needed: education, information, assistance and support. And that's exactly, what the book delivers«.

GETTING STARTED

Language is a strange thing. It does not matter which language; each has expressions that do not seem to make sense initially. One example is *irreversible*. There are few things left that really are irreversible; think judgments overturned or marriages dissolved by divorce. But when your doctor gives you an irreversible diagnosis, you should take it seriously. And here is where language starts to get funny: these diagnoses are usually called positive, even though the news itself is extremely negative. One infectious disease even is connected by name with the expression positive: HIV. What in the world could be positive about being diagnosed with an HIV infection?

The virus has been my constant companion for more than twenty years now. At the time I was diagnosed, the disease was a death sentence. Today, though still incurable, HIV is at least treatable. Nevertheless, today a positive HIV test result still is a cruel twist of fate, because probably no one is ever prepared for such a blow.

If you want to know how to live with the virus, you should ask a person who is infected. If you ever wondered how to lead a satisfying life with the virus, you should read this book. But beware: some long-cherished preconceptions may have to be abandoned. Nevertheless, this book does not contain a universal panacea. It gives insight into my story as well as my thoughts and feelings about the infection and what I have learned in the last twenty years. It is personal, it is subjective – and in a way it is also provocative. It gives an overview of the situation in Germany; some problems may differ from other countries, some problems certainly are similar. One thing is sure: a certain viral count in the blood is not yet a reason to die. There are so many ways to die, not only HIV. So let's get started with a retrospective and an optimistic look at life beyond HIV, beyond the virus.

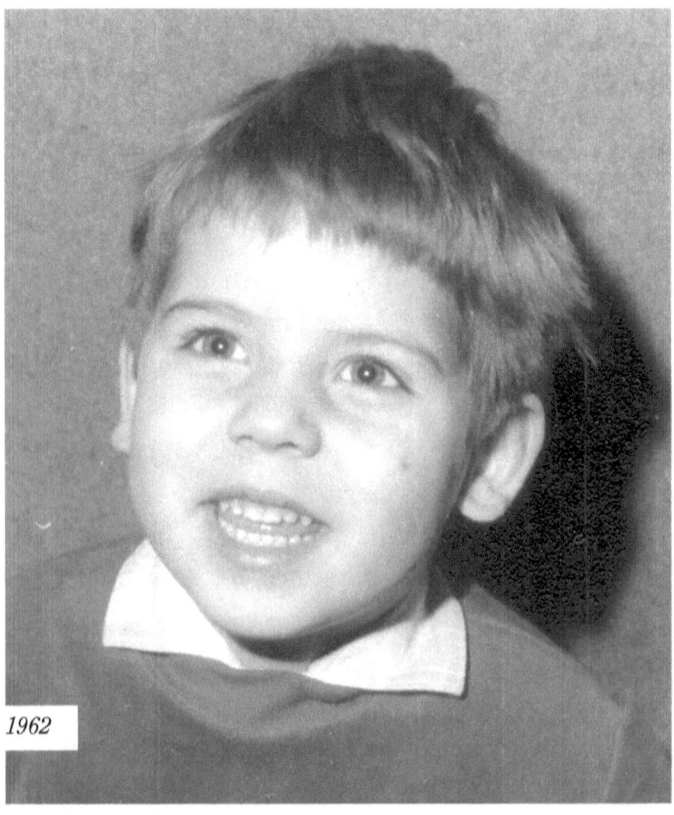

1962

GOING BACK IN HISTORY

I clearly remember January 1994 when I received my HIV diagnosis. At the time, I was freelancing for an independent TV-production company and had been working on three projects at the same time with twelve to fourteen hour days. I had been in Berlin for two years without seeing a doctor until I suffered from a general indisposition and abnormal fatigue, a medical condition that assailed me regularly when working too much. So I looked in the phone book and found a general practitioner around the corner. Even a thorough checkup did not show any noticeable problems. So the doctor decided to order complete blood work. When he was about to tap the vein, I turned my head and told him: »*Take a drop more and check the HIV status, too.*« He seemed a bit taken aback, but nodded silently and went on without further comment.

Actually, back then my asking for a HIV test was more surprising to me than the doctor. Although being part of a so-called risk group – I came out of the closet when I was twenty-three years old –, I had never checked my status before. It may sound strange, but I was as afraid of a positive result as of a negative one. The latter would have falsely proved that my half-hearted precautions for safer sex had been sufficient; or I had just been lucky. In fact, I never had given much thought about risk. Actually, I should have gotten the memo, when ROCK HUDSON, FREDDIE MERCURY and others died.

In Germany at that time, as elsewhere, gay sex was easy-going sex. There was no chance for pregnancy and if one caught a sexually transmitted disease, there was medication. That thoroughly changed in 1981, when first rumors about a new disease surfaced. Five young homosexual men in California considered healthy before, were suffering from a rare form of pneumonia. On July 3rd, 1981, the NEW YORK TIMES reported a »*rare cancer seen in 41 homosexuals*« – the Kaposi's sarcoma – which finally helped to spread the word of a »gay plague« all over.

The first infection was detected in Germany in 1982. One year later, the first German AIDS self-help group was founded in Berlin. The same year, ROBERT GALLO from the U.S. and LUC MONTAGNIER from France independently discovered a virus that would later be called HIV. Internationally, the first World-AIDS-Conference convened in Atlanta, Georgia in 1985, despite the travel restrictions imposed by the U.S. government on people with HIV or AIDS. In 1988, the United Nations declared December 1st as »World AIDS Day«. And since 1990, the Red Ribbon has been the worldwide symbol for the fight against the disease as well as the sign of solidarity and compassion.

But actually HIV is much older. The first proven infection was retroactively found in a blood sample of a Kenyan man taken in 1959. BETTY KORBER, a geneticist at the *Los Alamos National Laboratory*, dated the time of infection to 1931. In June 2008, MICHAEL WOROBEY, evolutional biologist at the *University of Arizona*, published research results about a sample taken in 1960, which dated the first transmission to between 1884 and 1924. Therefore it is doubtful that the five young men with whom ›modern‹ HIV history started in 1981 really were, as reported, completely healthy before. The diagnosed fungal pneumonia more likely resulted from an already existent immune weakness.

The first semi-official term for the disease was *Grid* (Gay related immune disease), colloquially called »gay plague«. In a 1982 White House press briefing, a journalist asked LARRY SPEAKES, spokesperson for President Reagan: »*Does the President have any reaction to the announcement by the Center for Disease Control in Atlanta, that AIDS is now an epidemic and has over six hundred cases?*« When the spokesperson responded: »*What's AIDS?*«, the journalist explained: »*It's called ›gay plague‹, too.*« Accompanied by a collective laughter Speakes replied: »*I don't have it. Do you?*« Later, to a question about whether the President or anybody in the White House knew about the epidemic, he had to admit: »*I don't think so*«.

The very same year the Robert-Koch-Institut, the *German Federal Institute for Infectious Diseases*, started to keep records on AIDS cases. Public opinion, however, simplified the danger of infection to three so-called risk groups: homosexual men, drug addicts and hemophiliacs. Especially gay men and drug users, groups historically already subject to discrimination, were deemed guilty of spreading the disease. In fact, gay sex life changed as the disease left a veil of sickness and death in the community. That made many men turn to safer sex only; some even renounced sex all together.

RITA SÜSSMUTH, at the time *German Federal Minister for Family Affairs, Senior Citizens, Women and Youth*, declared »*You do not get AIDS by chance, but by action*«. This meant everyone could shield himself from HIV by active self-protection, e.g. using a condom. And she really meant everyone, not only the risk groups. But the public turned the good idea behind the warning into the opposite. The second part of the recommendation, »*You get AIDS by action*«, was hijacked to imply that the sexual attitude of gay men inevitably led to HIV infection.

From then on German politicians, especially from the southern state Bavaria, demanded separating the sick from the healthy. In 1987 the German magazine DER SPIEGEL reported on the demand for mandatory registration and enforced survey of all citizens. This provoked the reproachful question of what to do with the infected people, once they were known by name. Terms like *final solution*, known from the Nazi times, popped up now and then. The Munich city councilman PETER GAUWEILER seized the opportunity to close gay bars, saunas and clubs to prevent the virus from spreading. Furthermore, he developed a catalogue of measures, which discriminated against gay men, drug addicts and prostitutes. Fortunately, it failed in most points; but the HIV test became a condition of employment, even for civil servants. Incidentally, the obligatory HIV test program was stopped in 1995 after the Bavarian state government had spent almost one million dollar on tests to find only four out of 78,400 being HIV positive. Back in 1987, a young, ambitious politician by the name of HORST SEEHOFER had pled unabashedly to »*concentrate HIV positive persons in special camps*«, though. By the way, he has been ›governor‹ of Bavaria since 2008.

Back to 1994. One week after the blood sample had been taken, I went to see the doctor again. Everything was normal except for one result. The doctor looked at me for a while, before he quietly asked:

»*Why did you want to know your HIV status?*«

»*I am part of a risk group*«, was my short, concise answer.

The doctor took off his glasses, rubbed his eyes and again looked at me with that glance that already told me what he was going to reveal.

»*You just get to know someone – and the first thing you have to do is to advise him of such a diagnosis*«, he said in a low voice. It was obvious that he did not want to say the word out loud.

If you are afraid of a negative test result, you should not be too surprised by a positive one. I was not surprised, but I was badly shaken. When the initial shock was over, I tried to deal with the situation and asked the doctor if there were any precautions I should take. My question was earnest. I did not have the slightest idea what lay ahead of me. The doctor's answer amazed me, especially the tone. He seemed to be close to tears:

»Enjoy your time left and make the best of it.«

I was sure I misheard the reply; I was bewildered. I did not intend to accept my fate without a fight and had hoped for some medical guidance. But now I did not dare to ask again. Nevertheless I stayed calm and tried to help the doctor over his solemn mood. Yes, indeed: I consoled the doctor.

After I left the doctor's office I was very sure I would never set a foot in it again. I was calm, but only externally. In fact, I was petrified and had not realized the implications of the news yet.

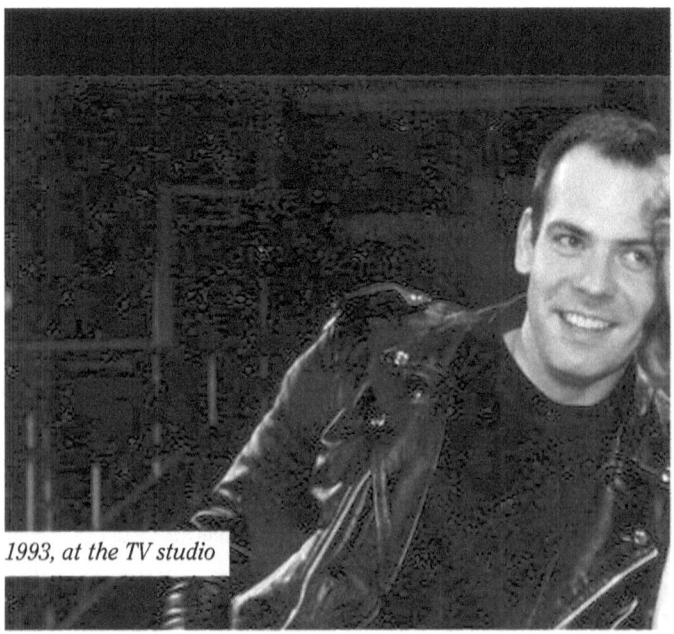

1993, at the TV studio

ANOTHER CLOSET TO COME OUT

It is not easy coming out of the closet, to admit being gay, as long as (still too) many people falsely believe homosexuality is a disease, a plague sent by God, or just the devil's work. But once you have decided to come out, your confidence in having done the right thing grows constantly. But if you are about to come out with an HIV infection, there is no guarantee whether it is the right thing to do at all. You cannot possibly deal with such a diagnosis by yourself. Some questions have to be evaluated very carefully: to whom/when/what and how much do I reveal? Should I talk about it at all? Do I know enough about the disease to answer inevitable questions? Can I cope with the comments? Possible reactions include sorrow, helplessness and consternation, revulsion, which can lead to bullying, discrimination, social exclusion or pure hate.

Let's get back to my story. After I left the doctor's office, I stood on the street for a while and took a deep breath. My irritation with the doctor's comment had dissipated; I had noticed that the doctor himself was shocked by the diagnosis he had had to reveal. So I got into my car and drove to the office. I needed to be back at the TV production company as I had no back up.

Working in a small unit, you quickly reach a more personal level with your colleagues. One of these colleagues,

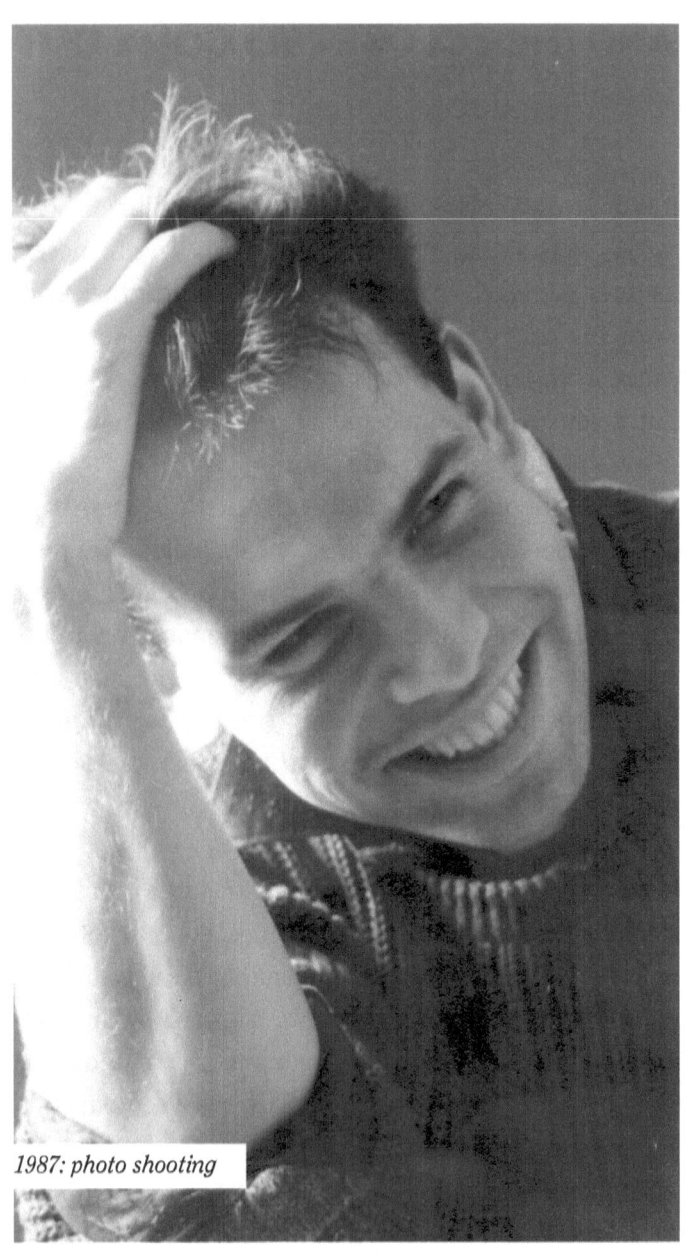

1987: photo shooting

the director's assistant, crossed my path shortly after I arrived at the office. She looked at me and addressed me in the usual way:

»Hey – you're looking strange!«

I shrugged and looked at her.

»Come on!«, she said and took me to her office, told me to sit down while she poured coffee into a mug. *»So – what happened?«*

I intended to answer: *»I just returned from the doctor«*. But at that very moment the tears I had been suppressing since the diagnosis erupted and I started to sob. On the way to the office, I had kept it together. But it had only been a front. I cried without restraint, stammering incoherent phrases, interrupted by sobbing and sniffling. Meanwhile, another colleague had entered the room, irritated by what he had seen through the open door.

Some minutes later my tears dried up; I straightened and took a deep breath. My colleagues exchanged glances before they looked at me. They had not yet had a chance to figure out, what had happened.

»I saw the doctor today. He checked my HIV status and the result is ›positive‹«, I blurted out.

»Shit!«. Just one word, but it hung in the room for quite a while. The colleagues' shock was patently visible. Already their first question was full of insecurity:

»How are we to deal with you now?«

»Please, no differently than before«, I replied. I had not changed; just something was wreaking havoc in my blood, something that did not belong there and would not go

away. This inalterable reality was hard enough for me to accept; how could my colleagues cope with it? Next, I informed the company's owner to preempt someone else telling him. I expected helplessness or statements of generic sympathy. But out of the blue, he asked: »*Do you want to change from freelancing to regular employment?*« I was astonished.

As a freelancer, I have no security whatsoever. I have to acquire jobs through my own initiative, take care of my own health and unemployment insurance, and have no claims to vacation or over-time. In short, I have no chance to benefit from any general labor laws. On the other hand, I am free to select assignments and carry out my own ideas, take the risk for their realization, and hopefully earn all the rewards, not only financial. Signing a regular contract would have given me some security. In 1994, nobody really knew about the future once you were infected. Except for death.

Although the offer was more than generous, I declined. It was my firm intention to go on as I had decided a couple of years ago: freelancing and successful. The owner respected my decision. His assistant however was stunned. I tried to explain my reasons to her, but she did not understand, or did not want to understand. My decision came from the gut. I still do not know whether I had wanted to prove my strength to myself or to others. But I have never regretted my decision. Not even more than twenty years later.

Coming out as HIV positive on the job is a decision that has to be considered very carefully. Today, in Germany not even thirty percent of the persons infected have done so. This is due to the unfounded, irrational fear of infection through daily contact prevalent in the general population. Actually it is discrimination against people who are somehow ›different‹. Also, it seems to be impossible to eradicate the false belief that infected people are less effective and motivated. And, last but not least, HIV positive people keep quiet in order not to expose themselves to potential bullying. Even in Germany, a country claiming to be progressive and enlightened, reactions to a coming-out as ›gay‹ are still unpredictable. That is why less than half of all homosexuals are out of the closet. However, an HIV infection confuses the issue. Thus those who actually are in the need of support and encouragement are left alone.

A German lawyer specialized in HIV related matters recommends not to reveal the infection in the workplace. Actually, it is not necessary to do so; the employer does not need to be informed until there is a severe effect on job performance, or a greater number of absences can be expected. Disclosure to one's employer can relieve pressure but opens the door to discrimination, rejection or even termination. The latter fortunately has been made impossible in Germany. In December 2013, the *German Federal Labor Court* officially recognized HIV as a disability according to the *German Federal Law for Equal Treatment* that prevents anyone from discrimination due to race, ethnicity, sex, religion or *Weltanschauung*, disability, age or sexual identity. Reason for the ruling was the dismissal of a 24-year-old lab assistant who disclosed his HIV infection prior to an announced official HIV test. In Germany, HIV infection falls under voluntary disclosure; no one is forced to reveal an infection, nor can anybody be forced to take an HIV test. In the named case, a pharmaceutical company requested a company-wide HIV test to protect employees and customers from a potential transmission of the virus. *Did they really mean to protect employees and customers?* Under the given circumstances, virus transmission at work was impossible. The lab assistant did not have customer contact. His task was to draw and control random samples during production, which were decontaminated afterwards. The hearing clarified an important point. Instead of dismissing the lab assistant, the company first should have checked if the workplace had suitable conditions for the HIV positive employee, or if accommodations could be made. Since the company had omitted to do that, the Federal Labor Court reverted the case to a lower court. In the final settlement, the employer admitted his omission. Nevertheless, the lab assistant was not interested in continued employment with the company, so he was granted severance pay.

Although there is no requirement to disclose HIV, my experience with being open about the infection has been good. All my friends and clients know; even my bank manager at the *Berliner Sparkasse* is in the know. So I was granted a loan a couple of years ago without any discussion. Moreover, in 2010, the bank published a story about me, about my disease and about my book in their customer magazine. For eight weeks my face appeared on every one of their twelve hundred ATMs in the German capital.

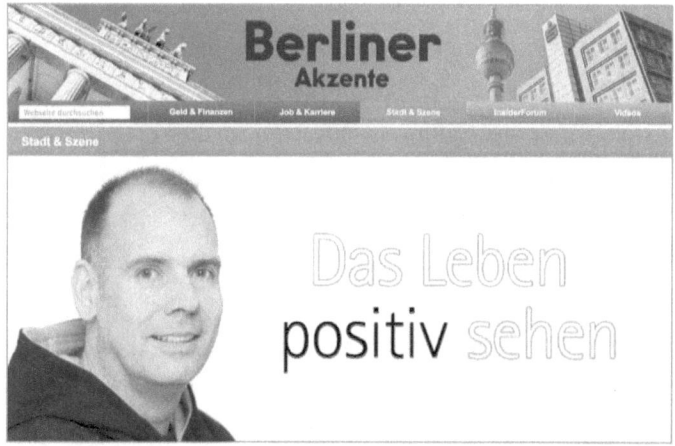

2010: »Das Leben positiv sehen« (Looking at life positively)
Cover story of the Berliner Sparkasse online magazine

I disclosed my infection to my colleagues more or less accidentally. Most likely, you would first tell your family or friends. My family is pretty large; I am the youngest of six children; we are very close though we live in different cities, and in one case, even on different continents. I am very close to my sister, who is five years older than me. So I called her the very evening of my diagnosis. I had overcome the initial state of shock and tried to look ahead. I had found out pretty quickly that there was no way to get rid of the virus, no matter how hard I tried. My sister's reaction was typical: silence and helplessness, but only in the first moment. Then she asked:

»What are you going to do now?«

»Actually, I have no idea. I have to get used to this thing first – and then need to think whom I am going to tell about it.«

»Who else knows about it?«

»Just three close colleagues, one of my clients – and you.«

»Do you want to tell our parents?«

Gee – that was a difficult question. In 1994, my parents were around seventy years old. They already had lost a child; my oldest brother died 1977 at the age of thirty from a cerebral tumor and I did not want them to grow older with the constant fear of losing their youngest child too early as well. Now two souls were dwelling in my breast: one asked me to have faith in the love and trust of my parents; the other one begged to keep any harm away from them. My sister preferred the latter: *»Don't tell them. They're pretty old now and presumably will die long before the disease will break out. Maybe there are treatments in the future. Who knows? If you tell them now, mum and dad will be worried sick to the end of their days.«*

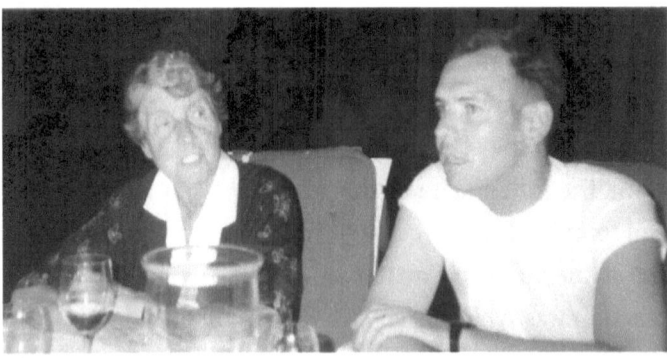

July 30, 1995, Weimar (Thuringia): My mom and me in a garden restaurant at my parents' 49th wedding anniversary

Touché. Good point. That made it easier for me to keep the truth to myself. But I never felt completely at ease with my decision. When my mom died six years later, my breach of trust became painfully wrenching. In the night before her funeral, I sat on the steps outside the church and cried; I would never be able to make it up to her.

My dad lived four more years; he died in 2004. We succeeded in concealing my infection from him, although one of my brothers almost spilled the beans. He had heard that I had had a medical checkup. And of all people, he asked my father whether there had been anything unusual. My father was quite upset and called me immediately. It took me some time to calm him down by explaining that I now had reached a certain age one has to take preventive checkups on a regular basis. So my parents were the only ones who never knew I was HIV positive.

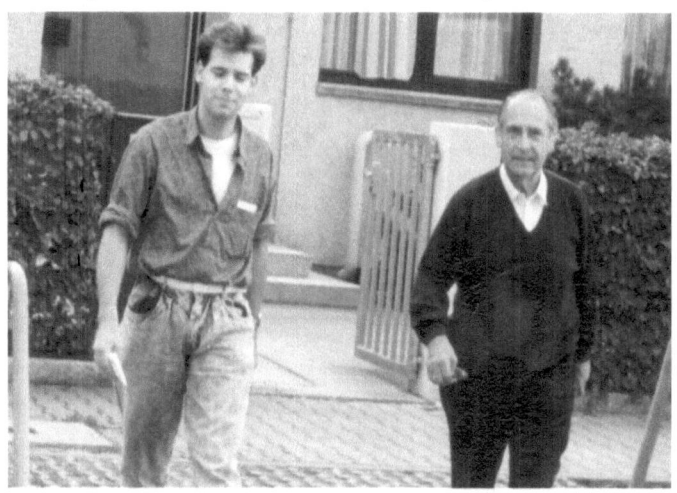

1988, Neu-Isenburg (near Frankfurt/Main): My dad and me in front of the company I worked for from 1984 until 1991

It did not take too long until I talked to the next generation. My nephews were eager to come to Berlin; they were twelve and thirteen years old on their first visit. I took them to the Olympic Stadium to watch a soccer game; we went to the movies and to restaurants. Later my niece arrived with a friend to paint the town. There were not too many places for sixteen year old girls to go on their own, but I showed them a couple of cool places they could boast about back home. Neither my brother and his spouse nor my sister had told them about my infection, but I thought they should know. So we talked about safe sex and HIV in general and my situation in particular. They were impressed by my frankness and honesty and felt taken seriously despite their youth. I guess, that is the only way to handle it.

Well, coming out on the job, with the family … what's next? My information hierarchy may differ a bit from the norm, since my friends were only third on my notification list, but that did not make them less important. In those days, my closest friend Thomas lived in Frankfurt/ Main. We had met about ten years earlier, when I also lived there. We remained close even after I moved to Berlin. But after my diagnosis, the telephone wire almost smoldered. A few weeks after the fatal date, I unexpectedly could take a couple of days off, which I wanted to use for a short vacation. Without further ado, Thomas decided to join me. So in March 1994, we went to the Turkish Riviera, exploring the area with a rental car, taking long walks on the deserted beach, talking intensively about everything but the

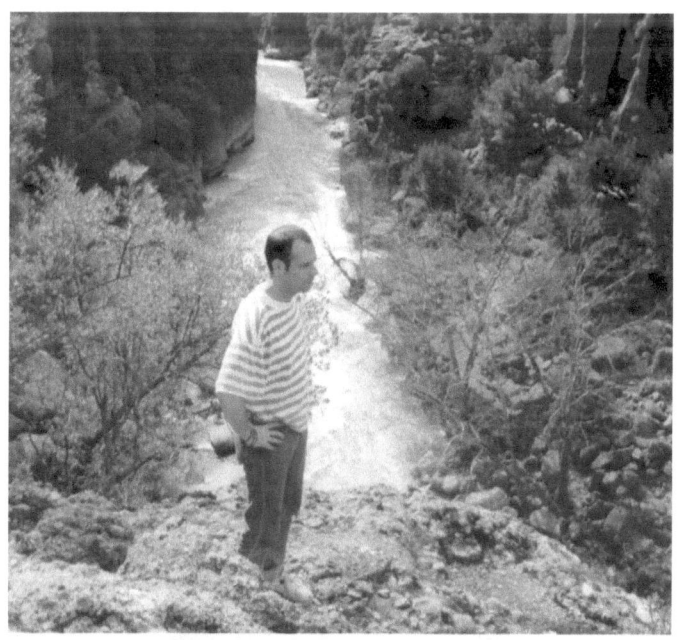

1994, Turkey: Mini vacation shortly after I received the diagnosis

kitchen sink, but mostly about me and my disease. Neither of us had an idea what would happen to me in the near or distant future, but we were sure we would master it somehow.

About one year later, I had more or less come to terms with my situation and accepted the infection as irreversible. This simplified how I handled it. What is accepted once, does not have to be questioned over and over again and there no longer is the need to constantly talk about it. I was on my way to some kind of normality, but Thomas was sure I was only deluding myself by suppressing the facts and the fears. I was irritated.

»How do you come up with that?«

»You're not talking to me. You can't avoid the disease!«
»Talking about it, makes it too important. The virus is part of me, not more. I don't want it to dominate my life.«
»You're not taking it seriously.«

That was the last straw: *»Of course I do. But I handle it differently than you would. There's nothing wrong with it!«*

»There sure is. I have no idea what to do if something happens to you!«

There you have it. I was silenced. How on earth could I have anticipated this reaction? It took me some time to respond. *»Well, Thomas, I don't know either. For me too, this is the first time I am HIV positive.«* Silence. We looked at each other. Suddenly a smile played on his lips, I could not fight a grin. Then we snorted with laughter.

With these positive experiences in mind I did not shy away from talking openly about my infection to friends or even business associates. Luckily, most of them commend my courage for handling HIV in daily life as positively as I do. There are two main reasons for my positive view: First, I was raised in a wonderful family of nine people: grandmother, mother, father and five elder siblings. My parents valued a good education and a strong personality. That eventually led to self-confidence and the development of verbal skills. The fact that musicality was (and still is) another widespread skill in our family, certainly pays off.

Secondly, I have learned a lot from my oldest brother, who died at the age of thirty. He suffered from a brain tumor that was discovered when he was fourteen years old (and I was one and a half years old). Within sixteen years,

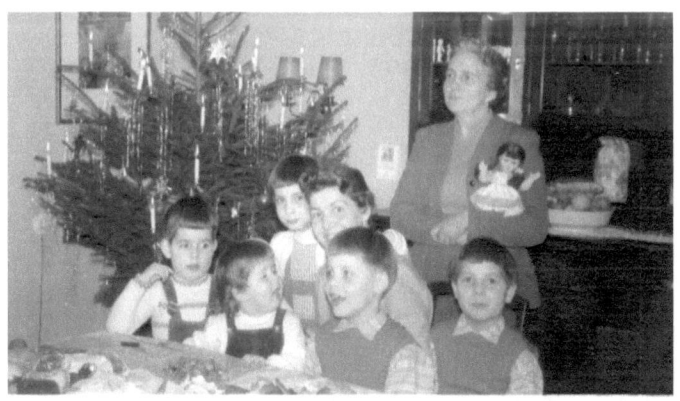

*Christmas 1958: My grandmother, my mom and
my five siblings ten months before I was born*

he endured five brain surgeries, but never lost his humor
and optimistic view of life. I very rarely heard him moan,
not even about the pain he must have suffered. I definitely took a leaf out of his book to handle my own life. So
when I got my diagnosis, I thought of him as an ideal.

I decide from case to case whether to tell people about
my HIV infection or not. If asked, I will not hide it.
Actually, nobody dares to ask. When I worked as press offi-
cer for a client at a film festival in France, I went out to
dinner with my colleagues, and as dessert I unpacked my
daily medication. I would have preferred to finish dinner
with a delicious *crème brulée*, but no chance. Instead I
noticed curious and bemused glances that I commented
with such general terms as *problematic hemogram, after-
math of a virus infection* or *metabolic imbalance*. That is
a wonderful aspect of HIV medication: you do not have to
be creative by inventing side effects. Just check the pack-
aging insert, there are plenty.

1999, Switzerland:
On top of the ›Schilthorn‹, a mountain 10,000 feet high

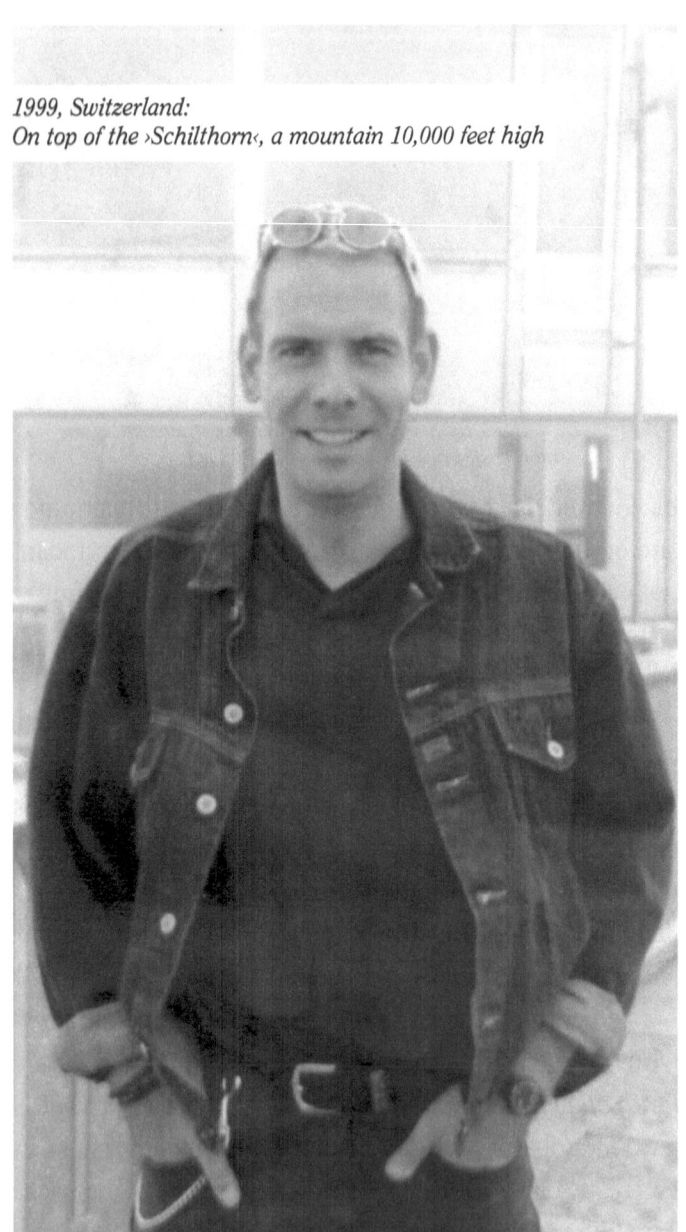

POSITIVE IN THE (GERMAN) GAY COMMUNITY

Worldwide 35.3 million people are infected with HIV, more than fifty percent of which are women and most likely not gay. *Well, so much for the gay plague.* Nevertheless, in Germany two thirds of the infected people are gay men. Gays also represent the largest percentage of new diagnoses. So: how does the gay community in Germany deal with HIV?

In the first years of my infection, my experiences in the gay community were varied and fall into three categories. Firstly, there were those being HIV positive themselves and thus feel called upon to be an honorary advisor: problem-oriented, extremely helpful and very sympathetic. Their desire to please me made me feel guilty that I was not in the mental crisis they thought I should be in and that they wanted to be able to untangle. Later, I noticed that most of them tried to solve their personal problems by offering a hand. Maybe this sort of support could help other people, but certainly not me.

Secondly, going out I came across men who preferred bareback (unprotected) sex once both partners had been tested positive. That was not my style. I believed (and still do) that there is the risk of a secondary infection by a different virus type or mutation. Up to now, there has been no proof of that risk, but no evidence makes me change my belief either. As long as this is not determined, I sympathize with the human immune system. What happens if the leukocytes, or later treatment, get confused which virus type they are to fight?

By the way: bareback sex today has lost a lot of its danger since studies have shown that the modern antiretroviral treatment reduces the viral load to the point at which the risk of infection is negligible, or even non-existent. Pre-exposure prophylaxis is yet a modern means of protection. Still, in my eyes, unprotected sex is like Russian roulette. You never can be sure if your partner is telling the truth about, or is aware of his HIV status, his actual viral load or whether he is in treatment.

And thirdly, there were those who broke off any contact when they heard about my HIV. Frightened or not, they just wanted to keep the topic as far away as possible. Or they had internalized the discriminating slogan »*Hands off of positive people!*«. Somehow I could understand that reaction. It was not what they said, but how they said it. Fear was something I might have been able to handle, but social rejection in terms of discrimination did hurt badly. And worse: this reaction came from the most interesting men. I ought to have known better. We are talking about a community that sets special value on externalities and is extremely youth-oriented. If you are in your mid-thirties and HIV positive, you are out. In the ›good old days‹ of personal ads as well as the successor internet the ideal hook-up was and is supposed to be aged eighteen to thirty-five – and healthy. When I turned thirty-six, I seemed to be out of the hook-up business anyway. But I was not too old for sexual encounters yet. Being honest about my health meant rejection, so only keeping the secret would help. But of course, keeping the secret meant safe sex only. I took sole responsibility for all actions pertaining to safety and preventing any risks. This unexpressed, unilateral obligation did not enhance pleasure at all, so I started to talk about the infection pretty early, even I risked of being turned down faster than I could vocalize the three-letter infection. Looking back at the last twenty years things luckily have improved at least in the major German cities. The »*No Chance for AIDS*« campaign, the many activities of AIDS self-help groups and activists have contributed to pull the disease out of the dimly lit, sordid corner. The public view has relaxed, and even when it comes to sexual contacts, my honesty is appreciated.

In many rural communities or very conservative areas however, HIV still is a no go. That is why it is so important to keep talking about HIV. Quite often I am confronted with arguments like, »*Why is there such a fuss about HIV, but not about cancer?*« Or »*Why is everybody asked to wear the red ribbon, but no one seems to care about multiple sclerosis?*« Exactly this shows how bigoted many people are. On the one hand, HIV is one of the very few incurable diseases from which you can actively protect yourself. On the other hand, it is often viewed as a self-inflicted disease, particularly when compared to the fateful diseases cancer or MS.

Alas, the best protection still is knowledge. This is exactly why I keep lecturing from my book, especially at school events. Learning about sexually transmitted infections is an important part of sexual education. And education helps to prevent infections and diseases in general. To date, I have held more than 200 lectures with questions-and-answers sessions and discussions afterwards.

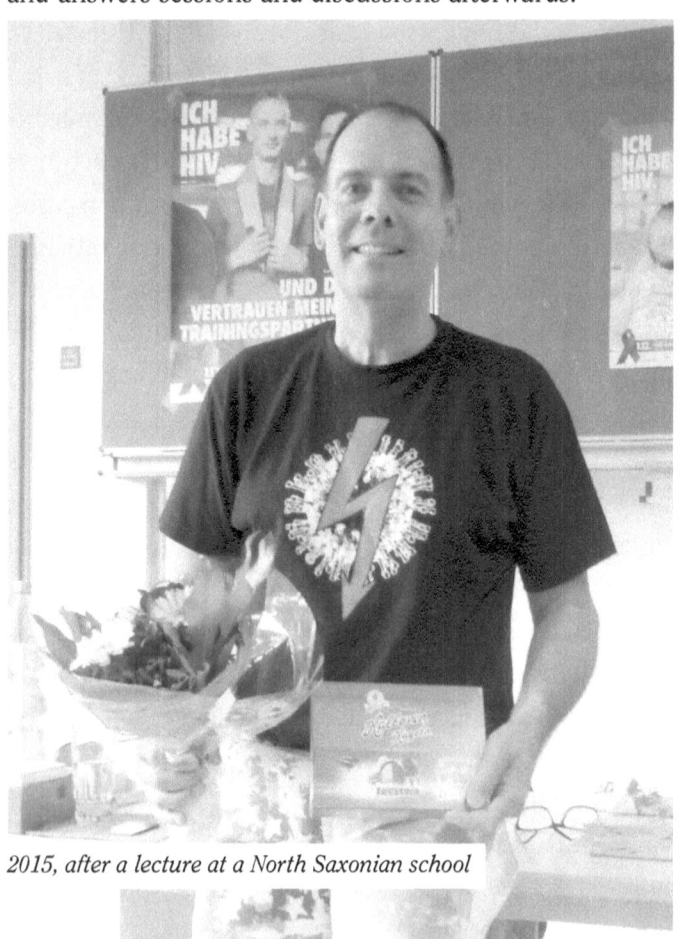

2015, after a lecture at a North Saxonian school

HOW DID IT HAPPEN?

The students in my lectures usually want to know how I got infected with HIV. And they want to know if I know who is to blame. As a matter of fact, I started to recall the potential situation fairly early and came across one night in Cologne 1992, shortly before I moved to Berlin. I had been out on the town and met a guy I liked. After flirting a lot and drinking even more, we decided to go to his place. I actually had already internalized the need for safe sex, but the alcohol reset all limits. I recall great sex that lasted until the birds began to sing. It had been a lot of fun, but thinking of the consequences, one has to ask if it was worth it. Nevertheless, I can't blame anyone except myself for disregarding all safe sex rules. By the way: blame or guilt are pompous words. They remind me of an index finger pointed at someone, indicating: *He's the one!*, which means nothing else than: *I'm not responsible!* But in my opinion, everybody is responsible for his actions, unless others take control or you abdicated from responsibility.

Students are confused when I tell them I do not feel hate or anger, and never tried to press charges against the guy. How could I? I moved to Berlin a couple of days later, and found out I was positive two years later. By then, I had forgotten the name and address anyway. And even if I pressed charges, or beat him up, or whatever, would that change anything about my HIV status? By the way, I am pretty sure, he did not know his status himself.

I have to add something about responsibility. Not only with gay sex, each partner is called upon to protect himself. Heterosexual men too often place the burden of responsibility for protection on women by expecting them to care for birth control. But as the name says, it is birth control and prevents unwanted pregnancy, but does not protect from venereal diseases or viruses.

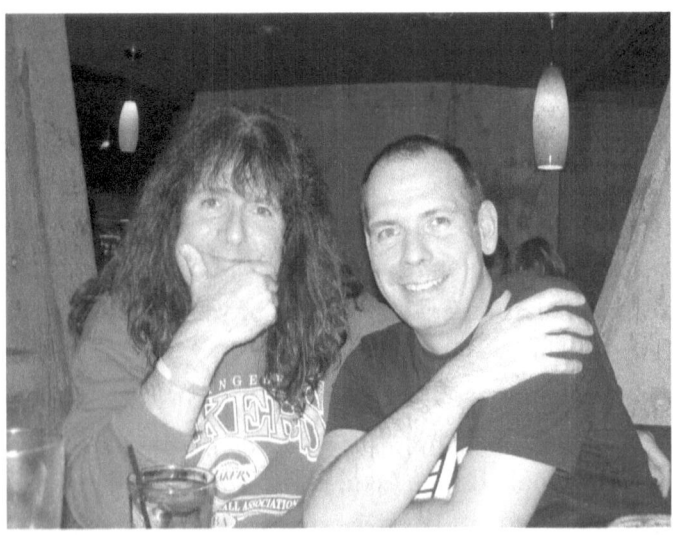

2006, Laguna Beach, CA:
Together with my brother Martin ›Martino‹ Gerschwitz,
who has been living in Orange County since the mid-80s.

ON MY WAY TO TREATMENT

First, let me apologize to the doctor who had the unhappy duty to inform me of my infection. Of course I felt offended by his statement: *»Enjoy your time left and make the best out of it«*, because it sounded like surrendering to the disease. I did not even think of this piece of advice as the only prescription a doctor could dispense in those days. Moreover, in my case, the doctor was a general practitioner whose patients mostly were senior citizens from the neighborhood. A gay and HIV positive patient in his thirties must have seemed an odd twist of fate indeed. So of course, he could not give advice on how to deal with the infection. In 1994, it was common knowledge that HIV eventually led to an early death.

As a matter of fact, the *»enjoy the rest of your life«* statement was quite prevalent until the mid-90s. Since there was no real effective cure or treatment for HIV, doctors often suggested to their patients to fulfill a last great wish. I have heard of people who quit their job, closed their accounts and sold everything they had to go on a cruise or world tour for several months. But I also have heard of people who came back and their state of health had not changed, not for the better or worse. But they returned flat broke and did not know where to go. That is the moment when you need friends. Friends who embrace you, find a job for you and let you know there is a future.

Sometimes I feel that in times of Facebook & co, friendship is not as highly valued anymore. A German proverb says: »*A friend is someone who takes you as you are.*« Another one reads: »*A friend does not ask. A friend does.*«

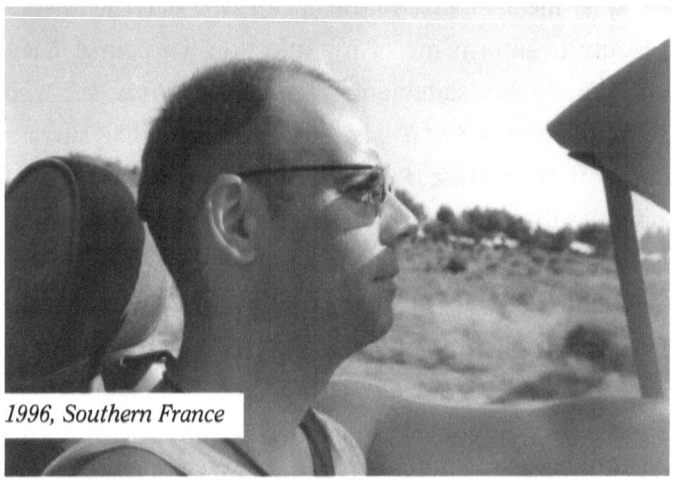

1996, Southern France

Before the diagnosis I never had wasted a single thought on what might come next. I always had thought this disease would never happen to me. So why should I have thought about the unavoidable consequences? The doctor's statement told me that I was beyond help. It was too late for precautions; so why should I ask for information? It may sound funny, but exactly this attitude prevented me from falling into a deep, dark hole. Not having the slightest notion what kind of harm the infection might do to me probably made me all the more determined to fight it mentally. I did not want to be beaten by a little virus! ›*Go and win!*‹, I said to myself. I was quite sure I would succeed even without a doctor ... at least without that doctor.

Two years went by without the need of any medical help. But in 1996 I finally had to see a doctor again as my stomach problems had become severe. The doctor was specialized in internal medicine, but with little HIV experience. She used every free minute to learn about HIV, for which I give her a lot of credit. She was flabbergasted when I told her I had not had a blood test since the diagnosis. She made up for lost time and checked the viral load. With an amount of 460,000 copies of the virus/ml blood, she suggested I start antiretroviral treatment immediately. My ears perked up: *antiretroviral what?* Obviously, the recent pharmaceutical progress had passed by me unheard. So I did not know that in 1996 antiretroviral treatment (ART), a triple combination of active agents, had been introduced. This was an apparent light at the end of the tunnel, but I refused her suggestion. I had found out that once I started with treatment, I would have to take the medication for the rest of my life, and I did not want to make such a major decision without a second opinion. She agreed.

Not long after I started a long-distance relationship with a guy living in the Ruhr area, some 500 kilometers (300 miles) away. My partner, as most of his friends, was also positive. They already were on the antiretroviral treatment, so I learned more about it up close. I did not like, what I saw. My boyfriend had to take six pills every four hours, even at night – up to 36 tablets a day. That certainly was not my piece of cake.

My next blood test showed a viral load of 51,000 copies, which meant, the viral load had decreased by ninety percent. Again my doctor suggested starting with treatment. Having seen, how friends dealt with treatment, I refused once more. Instead of telling her the true reasons, I suggested a deal: »*Let's wait another three months. If the viral load again has decreased, this time below the limit of detection* (1996: 50 copies/ml, 2015: 10 to 20 copies/ml blood), *you will stop to practice, I quit my job too, and the two of us will be stars in all the TV talk-shows: you as the quack and I as the wondrously healed patient.*« I loved the idea, but of course it didn't work. Three months later my viral load had gone up 110,000 copies. Pity, too much for TV shows. But I still refused treatment.

In 1998, a friend recommended his doctor, who practiced at a center for infectious diseases. At this time common practice was to start treatment only when the immune system really needed help, which was determined by the number of T helper cells. As there were few agents available, starting treatment too soon could have caused the virus to become resistant, leaving no alternative agents. On the other hand, the newly improved pharmaceutical products allowed smaller and less frequent doses: only two or three times per day. I felt comfortable with this approach as well as with the doctor. For the next two years, I had my blood checked every three months with no abnormalities.

In 2000, events escalated so that I could not to keep up with the regular checkups. In May, completely unexpected, my mother was diagnosed with end-stage cancer. My father was not too healthy, either; he just had been classified to care level one. This means he benefitted from in home assistance for a few hours daily granted by the German social security system because he was limited in taking care of himself. So additionally my siblings and I rotated taking care of our parents. They lived some 550 kilometers (350 miles) from Berlin

Two months later, my boyfriend at the time, who lived 850 kilometers (530 miles) away in Switzerland, ended our relationship. As I spent every spare moment with my parents, I could not travel to Zurich or see him in Berlin often; our relationship was reduced to telephone calls. He felt placed on the waiting list. And anyway, he had problems with the geographic distance separating us. This new situation was too much for him.

My mother finally died in late August. Two weeks later I was informed that my main assignment for the TV production company I had been working for since 1995 would end in six weeks. And there was no follow-up in sight. I was nearly bankrupt.

The stress that had lasted for months, the losses and the insecure financial situation took their toll. Now I could have gone back to the regular health checks, but I feared the worst and did not want to take another blow. But reality could not be ignored.

My professional situation improved by November with a prospective long-term freelancing job in the movie industry. But it took until February the following year for me to see the doctor again. Unfortunately, my apprehension was confirmed: my blood values had changed for the worse. The viral load had gone up and the helper T cells had decreased dramatically. Treatment was now inevitable. Considering I had not been too careful with my health in the last few years – smoking, drinking and partying excessively – my health had held up pretty well.

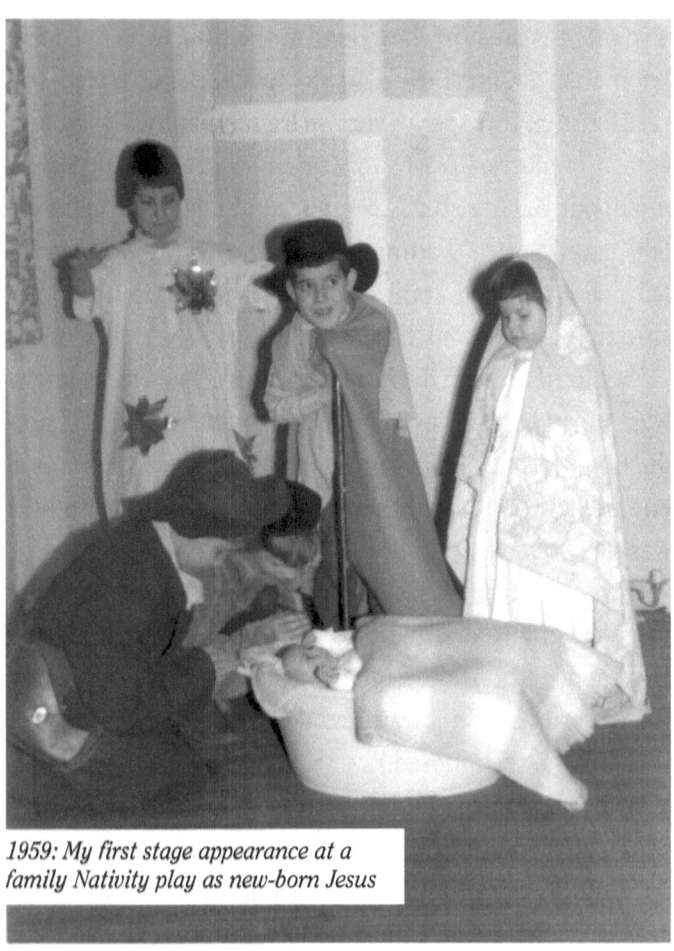

1959: My first stage appearance at a family Nativity play as new-born Jesus

A POSITIVE ATTITUDE
IS A GOOD START

I do have fond memories of the early 80's, when the expression »positive« meant something really positive, i.e. good. In those days, a radio station in southwestern Germany broadcasted a humorous little forty second-feature every morning called »*Health training for healthy people*«. This feature was meant to let the listeners begin the day in a good mood. Every show started with the same phrase: »*Start your day positively*«, which soon became a well-known expression, until the day, when the *positive* got a second, fatal meaning through HIV and AIDS. The show was taken off the air.

But why? There are more meanings of positive than just the medical one. Actually, the feature intended to influence the mind. Popular wisdom has it that a positive attitude towards life fosters health and has beneficial effects on treating depression. There is even a proverb saying »*laughter is the best medicine*«.

A study from the UNIVERSITY OF TEXAS a couple of years ago found out that a positive attitude towards life can even delay the process of aging. It can do the very same for dealing with an incurable illness, even if the illness is called positive, too. You just have to let it happen.

The attitude towards life is what separates the optimist from the pessimist. I claim to be incurably optimistic. I carry the secret probably in my genes, or as the German poet laureate JOHANN WOLFGANG VON GOETHE (1749 – 1832) put it: »*I inherited stature and serious approach to life from my father; from my mother however, the cheerful nature and delight in telling stories*«.

But when it comes to what optimism really can effect, I gladly remember my eldest brother. As I wrote before: he died 1977 a few days after his thirtieth birthday as a result of a cerebral tumor he suffered from for sixteen years. He

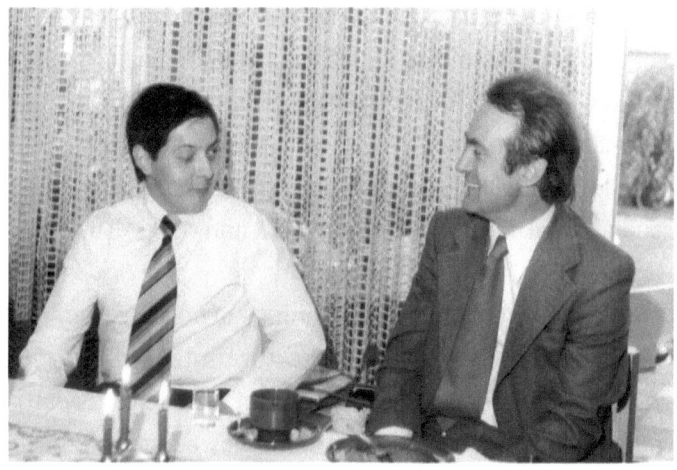

1976: my eldest brother Christoph (1947 – 1977, on the left) together with Johannes Rau (1931 – 2006), a friend of the family who 1999 was elected Federal President of Germany

had endured five brain surgeries, but never lost his humor and optimistic view on life. When I turned thirty in 1989, I dedicated that special day to his memory. Still today, I am very thankful for all I learned from him – and it's not only his optimism.

I have been asked quite often if my positive way to handle HIV is genuine or just a front. If one is raised as close to illness as I was, then illness somehow becomes normal and, oddly enough, becomes less threatening. That is not to trivialize HIV, but more or less the one and only way to handle it: if you cannot beat it, live with it.

Inevitably that leads to confusing situations. Being equipped with unshakeable optimism, I take life in a stride. Sometimes people who do not know me may think I do not take life seriously enough. You remember the dispute with my best friend Thomas a couple of pages ago? He accused me of ignoring reality while I tried to tell him that I would not let the virus get the better of me – and of my life. Additionally, I really do love the German language with all its linguistic potential, even when it comes to the infection. One of my favorite phrases translates as follows: »*Deep down in my heart I have always been a positive person. Why shouldn't the body follow suit?*«

When it comes to phrases like that, there are two opinions. Some laugh and accept that I take HIV with a smile; others accuse me of lacking earnestness, which of course is not true. Even more: how much earnestness is needed to live a good life? Aphorisms like the one above free me from handling HIV and facilitate others handling me. It is true indeed: laughter is the best medicine. It is a pity there are too many people around who obviously are not receptive to teasing.

The effects of pessimism on life were also one of the reasons that ended the relationship with my Swiss boyfriend. Due to the distance, we met more or less every three weeks for a couple of days, mostly in Zurich. With him, the joy of being together again soon mixed with the sadness of my inevitably upcoming departure. So he was never able to savor the shared moments to the fullest. I on the other hand enjoyed every single minute of the shared time. Although every goodbye was difficult for me too, I already focused on the next reunion. With such a constellation, a relationship is doomed. Presumably, we should have known better beforehand. When it comes to real feelings, you think you are strong enough to overcome these differences. But soon reality gains ground, and you are standing in your own way. The result: Murphy's Law, »*Anything that can go wrong, will go wrong*« proves itself again.

A pessimist stands in his own way, and fails to appreciate good fortune. An optimist, however, does not count setbacks as defeat, but as a chance to rejoice even about the tiniest bit of good fortune. And good fortune definitely is something to honor. The great French philosopher VOLTAIRE (1694 – 1778) put it in a wonderful phrase: »*Since it is beneficial to my health, I have decided to be happy.*«

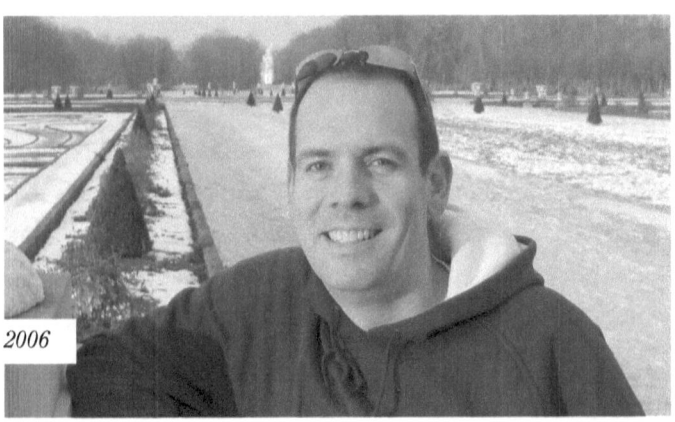

2006

THE DAILY DOSE

HIV patients are not the only ones on earth who have to take medication regularly, but it is the size and the color of the pills that reminds me more of candy than of health. But they do not taste nearly as good. Luckily since 1996 there is effective medication to keep the virus in check. To be honest: I am extremely happy that the effective medication was found shortly after my infection was detected. Even if it took me some years before I started with treatment.

Until 1987, there was nothing but illusory hope, sickness, sorrow, mourning and death. Then the Federal Drug Administration (FDA) approved an agent called »azidothymidine« or AZT for HIV treatment. This agent had been developed in 1964 to fight cancer, but never succeeded. With HIV it seemed to be able to stop the virus spreading in the body. Admittedly, AZT had to be administered in a high dosage, which caused a lot of side effects and quite a few patients succumbed to these. This led to the false impression that it was the medication that killed people, and not the virus. Even today there still are some doubters who will never be convinced and continue to subscribe to this outdated opinion.

When antiretroviral treatment (ART) was introduced 1996 at the Vancouver World Aids Conference, everything changed. With ART (sometimes HAART = Highly Active

Antiretroviral Treatment) the effectiveness of the medication eclipsed the deadly side effects. Already in 1997, the Centers of Disease Control (CDC) reported a decrease in HIV/AIDS related deaths for the first time. But even with ART, patients have to cope with inconveniences.

Starting with treatment means suddenly feeding the body with agents it is not used to. A stomach in revolt is the smallest evil. It takes about two weeks until the metabolism gets used to the regular doses of medication; but that does not mean all functions of the body normalize again. Stomach problems, headaches and indigestion are daily occurrences; much worse is the diarrhea, especially when it comes without warning. I remember days when I had to plan trips around Berlin very carefully to ensure a public or private toilet could be found at short notice. In those days, I developed the dictum, if you will pardon my saying so: »*Diarrhea is shit*«. Fortunately, a change of medication at least spared me from that evil. But there is more: abnormal fatigue, lightheadedness and insomnia. Sometimes neuralgia in arms and legs occurs; a dysfunction of the lipid metabolism up to lipodystrophy may cause fatty tissue to shift from the face, arms or legs to the abdomen and/or neck.

Treatment has effects on the psyche, too. After the diagnosis there is a vague hope to at least mentally vanquish the pathogens. But eventually the day comes when the viral load has significantly increased and the number of T helper cells has decreased substantially. Now the immune system needs help. Starting treatment means the psychological battle has been lost. This is a dramatic milestone, probably even more dramatic than the diagnosis itself. I have met quite a few people who showed changes in personality after starting treatment; not at all for the better. They made decisions nobody could understand or ended long friendships without reason. I had friends who had run an open house, parties, game nights, Sunday afternoon *cheesecake teatime*, but when both of them had to start treatment, they literally closed the doors and windows. Others, who were real workaholics and loved their profession, suddenly decided to quit and live on a disability pension.

German pension funds allowed the early retirement for HIV patients up to the end of the 90s. The reason was simple: HIV reduced life expectancy considerably and thus those infected would not burden the system for too long. But since antiretroviral treatment has improved both the quality of life and increased the life expectancy, the early retirement program was stopped. Only my disability pass, granted in 2001, is left. The pass provides some advantages, including cut-rate entrance fee for my favorite soccer team *Hertha BSC Berlin* and a tax allowance of around $1,000 per year.

Some of those whose life had changed with the treatment have managed to gain ground again. Others could not come out of the deep dark hole they had fallen into even with helping hands. Conversely, treatment can have positive effects, too: a friend told me that soon after he started taking the pills his mental well-being as well as his physical performance had steadily grown. My personal experience: until now, I have managed to overcome phases of listlessness and lack of motivation. And the feedback I receive at readings and lectures keeps me upbeat.

The side effects alone should be enough to deter from getting infected at all. True, treatment has positive results: regaining quality of life and increased life expectancy. It seems young people are under the false impression that pills cure HIV. But they don't. I remember people saying in earlier days: »*HIV positive? Leave me alone! I don't want to swallow pills for the rest of my life.*« Today I often notice a kind of indifference: »*If it happens, it happens. Thank God, there is treatment.*«

I am flabbergasted people think this way. I am very grateful for the medical progress of the last twenty years, but just because there is treatment does not mean you cannot get infected. Death remains a part of HIV and AIDS. In Germany, around 750 people die each year as a consequence of the infection.

Today it seems quite normal to take pills for everything: for fun, for sleep, for happiness, for virility and lots of other (frivolous) reasons. Obviously, we are used to a certain *pill mentality*. Getting infected with HIV seems to be collateral damage. I profoundly disagree with this development. My experience from more than twenty years with the infection and over fifteen years of steady medication and side effects: A life without HIV certainly is the better choice.

GOOD NEWS ABOUT
THE TREATMENT

There is a simple reason why the antiretroviral treatment is always called an effective medication: it works! Otherwise my health insurance would not incur the $45,000 expense per year for medication prescribed due to the infection. But actually how does the treatment work?

The threat of HIV always has been that the virus would spread in the body by invading the healthy cells of the immune system, transform them into HI virus production cells and send the newly produced HI viruses out to invade more healthy immune cells. This continues until the immune system collapses completely. Then even harmless infections can be fatal. This is the theory; in practice, it takes years without treatment until the immune system collapses. But it sure will do.

The antiretroviral treatment concentrates on controlling HIV by interrupting the process of invading immune cells and their multiplication. The medication blocks the receptor or, literally speaking, the entrance to the immune cell. Since the HI virus, as a retrovirus, needs a host cell to survive, the viral load decreases slowly but steadily as the receptors are blocked and the viral load falls below the detection limit. However, some virus cells survive in so-called reservoirs to which the medication does not yet have access. That is why, to date, HIV cannot be completely eliminated and still is incurable.

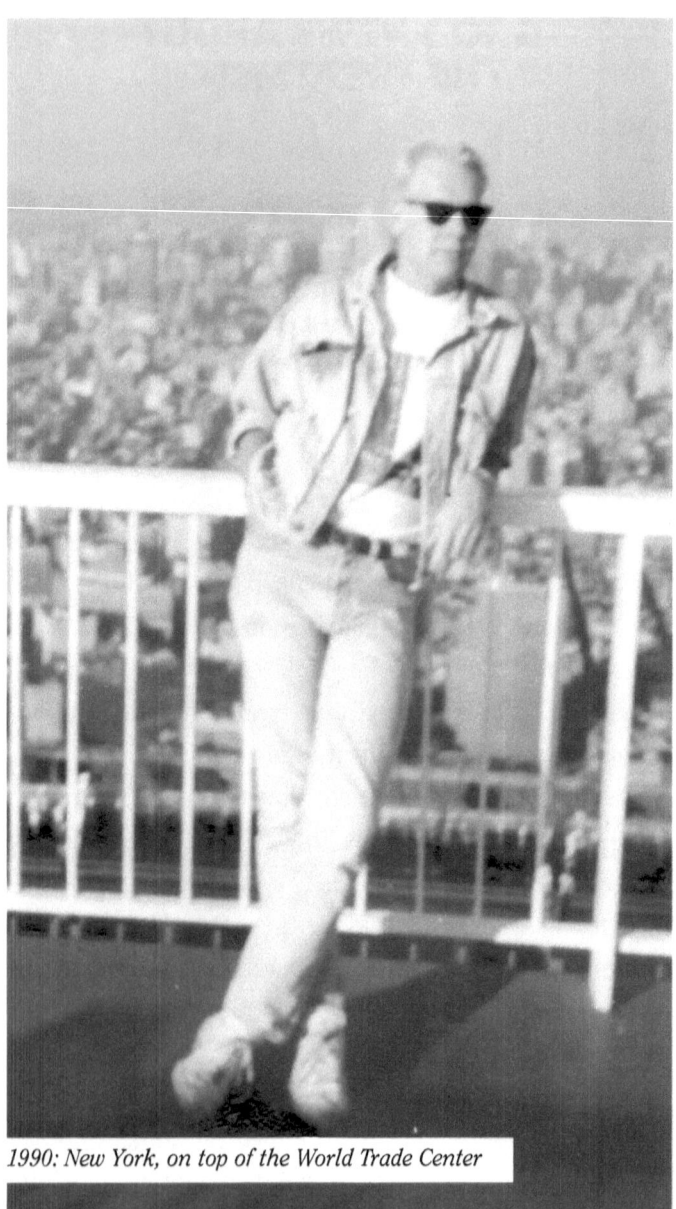

1990: New York, on top of the World Trade Center

But a viral load as low as under the detection limit is a great step forward. First of all, it ensures that the virus no longer threatens the immune system. Secondly, it reassures people in one's direct environment they need not fear transmission. Actually, they never had to, as long as there was no direct exchange of blood or any other infectious body fluid. Insufficient knowledge of HIV causes many people to feel at risk in situations when they really are not. The risk is in their mind only. A little initiative to get information could space them that. In this respect unfortunately little has changed.

There is one thing HIV negative people have not understood yet: a certain viral load is needed to transmit the disease. Once you take the antiretroviral drugs, the viral load sinks below the detection limit and, consequently, transmission is highly unlikely if not impossible. In 2008, the Swiss AIDS-Commission published a startling statement:

»HIV infected persons on effective antiretroviral treatment (and free of other STDs) are sexually non-infectious. Having taken into consideration all scientific evidence, the Expert Clinical Commission on HIV/AIDS Treatment of the Federal Office of Public Health, and after great deliberation, the federal committee for issues related to HIV/AIDS has arrived at the following conclusion: HIV seropositive individuals on antiretroviral treatment with a fully suppressed HIV viral load (hereafter referred to as ›fully suppressive antiretroviral treatment‹) and no additional sexually transmitted infections do not transmit

HIV by sexual means. This assertion is contingent on the following conditions:

- *That the HIV+ individual is under the care of a treating physician and that s/he takes the medication exactly as indicated;*
- *That the HIV viral load is below the level of detection of common viral load tests (>undetectable<) and has been for at least 6 months;*
- *That the HIV+ individual is not currently experiencing any other sexually transmitted infections.«*

This statement aimed at partnerships with partners of different HIV status, so-called serodiscordant partnerships. But it applied only if the negative partner had been thoroughly informed and had consented.

In the same year, a Washington D.C. Aids specialist told GQ magazine that after six months of treatment no active virus was found in sperm or blood. After two years of treatment the danger of transmission was practically nonexistent. It took some time for official authorities to agree. Today HIV research has come to the conclusion, that antiretroviral treatment prevents transmission by ninety-six percent, if the conditions of the Swiss statement are fulfilled. Nevertheless, my personal opinion is that the negative partner is the only one to decide if protection is necessary.

But treatment has shown side effects in addition to the ones named previously. Doctors noticed an increase of comorbidities: an HIV infection can facilitate the transmission of other infectious diseases, especially hepatitis. And the treatment itself increases the risk of cardiac arrest and stroke. This is why regular checkups are essential for HIV patients. But weighing advantages and disadvantages, the treatment certainly is the best way to handle HIV.

Since treatment demonstrably improves the health of HIV infected people, UNAIDS, the Joint United Nations Program on HIV/AIDS, launched ambitious new targets to scale up of antiretroviral treatment in 2014, known as »90-90-90«:

– By 2020, 90% of all people world-wide living with HIV will know their HIV status.
– By 2020, 90% of all people with diagnosed HIV infection will receive sustained antiretroviral treatment.
– By 2020, 90% of all people receiving antiretroviral treatment will have viral suppression (a viral load below the detection limit).

Only one year later, at the *8th IAS Conference on HIV Pathogenesis, Treatment and Prevention* held in Vancouver 2015, experts presented demoralizing statistics: while European countries and Australia already have come close to meeting the target, especially the United States falls far short of reaching them. According to a US survey done in 2013, 86% of the people living with HIV know about their status; that's almost 90%. But only 37% of them receive sustained antiretroviral treatment, a far cry from the 90%

targeted. And barely 30% of those receiving antiretroviral treatment, instead of UNAIDS's visionary target of 90%, show a viral load below the detection limit. This is a very poor performance for the country that faced the first cases of the epidemic in 1981. Only four out of thirteen monitored countries or regions showed worse results in general: Sub-Saharan Africa, Georgia, Estonia and Russia. There is a lot of work left to be done.

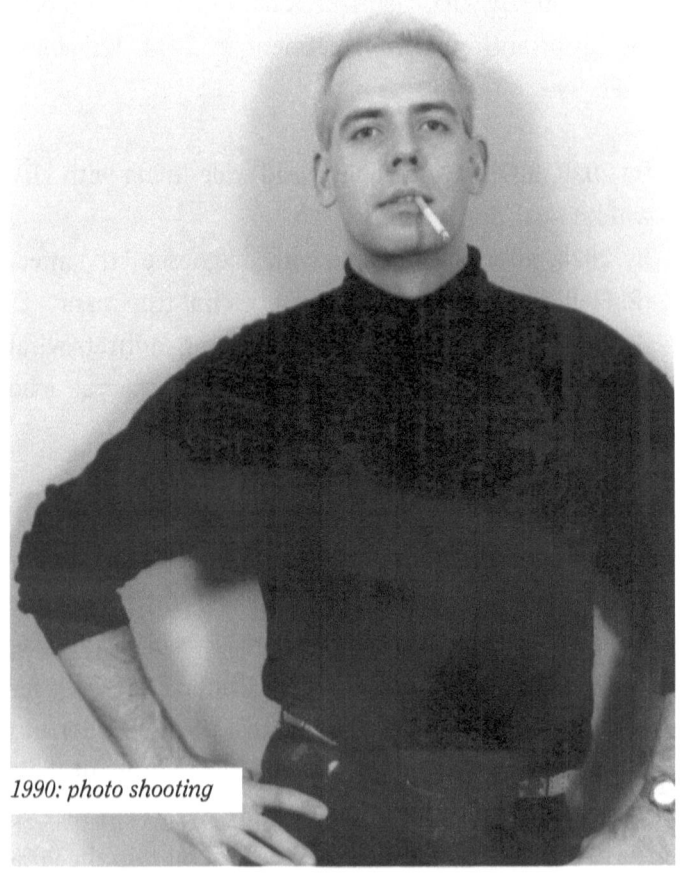

1990: photo shooting

IN THE LONG RUN
WE'RE ALL DEAD

I have friends who tend to get sad about the fact that I will die. Of course they are right, but I usually tell them that they cannot cheat death either. I remember in the 70s there was a German saying that translates to »*Life is one of the hardest and usually ends with death.*« The wisdom in this expression has not changed within the last forty-five years.

Of course I appreciate the intention of empathy and sympathy. I have been living with HIV for more than twenty years now, and have been living pretty well with it. But in all these years was I confronted so often with statements like: »*But HIV is incurable!*« I know that already ... so what's new?

My existence does not only circle around HIV. There is so much more to life! And I am doing well! This kind of sympathy actually focuses on the disease instead of me. The virus is not half as interesting as I am, especially with a viral load under the detection limit. Let's not talk about diseases all the time, not even the one I have. There are so many things I prefer to do or I want to learn about. HIV is just a fact. Not less, but not more either.

Nevertheless, it happens, whether I want to or not. As HIV positive you have to develop a thick skin not to be crushed by the accumulated weight of sympathy. So please remember: the best and most important support is not sympathy, but interest in my life; to learn and to understand, and to fight ignorance. And I ask for nothing less than acceptance, or at least tolerance, to fight discrimination and stigmatization. Just treat me (and others) the way we are, do not wrap us in cotton wool. Just be as considerate to us as to all others. Or, as the German writer FRIEDRICH HEBBEL (1813 – 1863) once said: »*Nature gave many a talent for sympathy, but only a few are talented for sharing joy.*« If it comes to me, I would go in for sharing the joy of life.

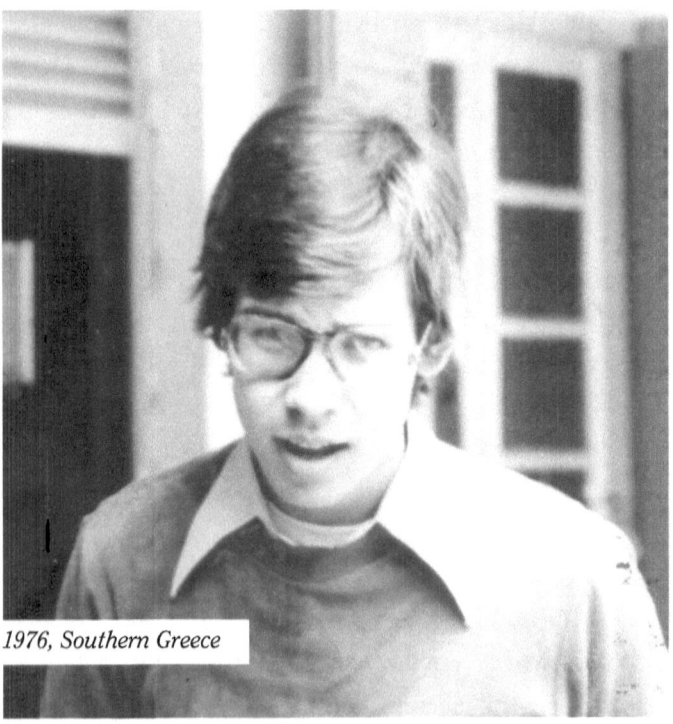

1976, Southern Greece

FATE OR GUILT?

Sometimes you are confronted with the oddest situations. For about ten years I worked for different TV production companies, organizing and taking care of the talk-show studio audiences. I remember one production titled »*How to deal with incurable illness*«. The editorial staff had put together a group of six people with various diagnoses: breast cancer, lung cancer, brain cancer, diabetes and two HIV positive men. The audience consisted of people affected, members of self-help groups, patient organizations and social service professionals. The guests also had brought family members and friends. Technically, and in terms of content, the taping went well; the sensitive moderator ensured that the show was profound and informative. As soon as the cameras were switched off and the guests had left the stage, a storm of protest broke out. Relatives of the cancer patients attacked me for daring to combine cancer and HIV on the same stage. I pointed out that this had been an editorial decision. When I said, there was no reason to take issue with the content, the protests escalated to new heights. I then was accused for having lured cancer patients and their relatives and friends onto the show under false preconditions, and placing them, without warning, next to a *bunch of gay guys*.

I tried to understand, but somehow couldn't. Were they afraid of being infected by just sitting together? Or did they really believe cancer was fate and HIV was a self-inflicted disease only afflicting gays? I did not have to wait for long to hear that statement again: »You do not get AIDS by chance, but by action« But this time it was not only a general reproach, it was a cynical accusation made by relatives of incurably sick people towards relatives of likewise incurably sick people.

The companions of the two HIV positive men overheard the comment. They demanded an apology for the verbal assault, but nothing happened. A dispute ensued which quickly became very ugly. Every attempt to talk sense failed. So I threw all of them out of the studio.

I could not stop thinking about the incident all night. I had never experienced anything like that. I had intentionally not revealed my HIV status because I did not want to be seen to take sides. Still the insults hit me personally, too. So the next day I decided to write a letter to all parties requesting them to reflect on their behavior. Furthermore, I challenged them to tell the difference between a correct sickness like cancer and an incorrect sickness like HIV. Of course, I demanded an apology to the other party for their verbal attacks. I actually received some half-hearted apologies, which I passed on.

Although this experience was many years ago, I still cannot understand what motivates people to display that sort of unkindness. Unfortunately, that has not changed. No one has ever been able to tell the difference between a valid and an invalid disease, not then, not now. But to be honest: I had not expected an explanation of the distinction anyway. Hopefully, it made those people think. With incurable diseases there is no correct or incorrect, no good or bad, no better or worse. There is only understanding and compassion, assistance and support. And, of course, hope. That, at least for me, is the only way to seriously and caringly deal with the sickness of another person and its consequences.

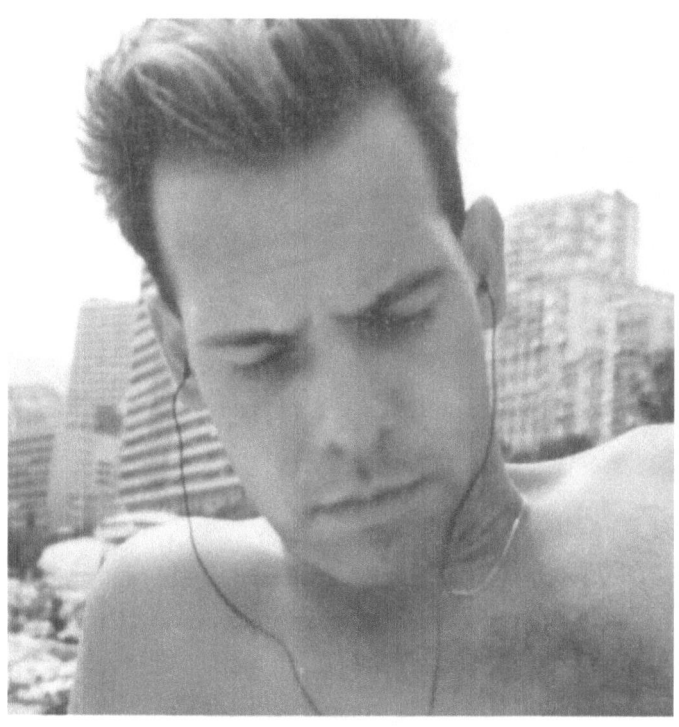

1988, Montecarlo Beach

DREAM A LITTLE DREAM
OF ... PROTECTION

Actually it is so easy to protect oneself from any venereal disease, including HIV: just use a condom! But throughout its existence, the little protective device never has been all that popular. Back in my youth in the 1970s and 80s, dealing with sex had become more relaxed than in the decades before. The sexual revolution in Germany of the late 60s/early 70s had socially contributed to what the pharmaceutical industry had medically set in motion. The birth control pill made sexuality carefree by protection from unwanted pregnancy. And for STDs there was penicillin. Despite the openness about sex, buying condoms was embarrassing in those days. But did you know there was a celebrity who trusted condoms? The world renowned Italian seducer, GIACOMO CASANOVA (1725 – 1798) is known to have used condoms made from sheep's intestine to protect himself from the at his time rampant syphilis. Very clear-sighted, you may say. Isn't Casanova the best testimonial a condom could have? If he was able to enjoy his pleasure with protection, why are today's men afraid condoms might diminish it? Even after 1981, when HIV and AIDS first appeared, and sexual transmission was considered the main threat, only sex without a condom was considered proper and manly. It certainly looked like a rebirth of the Neanderthal man, whose main occupation was hunting animals, collecting food and defending wife and hearth.

But ten thousands of years after this sapient, and some two hundred years after Casanova, today's males obviously are not as tough as their ancestors. The reasons for rejecting condoms remain the same. Condoms come between two people having intercourse, their usage interrupts intercourse because you have to stop to put one on, and they generally reduce desire. Or think of the infamous latex allergy, which could lead to itching and erythema, and even anaphylactic shock!

Caution!

Irony!

Well, there are products made of hypoallergenic latex, but that solution is probably too easy. Or men were afraid that a German comic called »*Condom of Horror*«, published in 1988, might come to life? The book's illustrator, RALF KÖNIG, has a condom armed to the teeth bite off man's best part, thus leaving a bloody trail of horror.

Actually, the attitude towards condoms mirrors the time. With all the pharmaceutical and social progress, liberal sexual behavior became quite prevalent for the young generation of the 70s. You could talk about sex freely and experiment without embarrassment, and the more the better. Gonorrhea could be a status symbol as it was proof of a very active sex life. Why should that attitude change after the arrival of HIV and AIDS? That was something that afflicted gay men, so heterosexuals were not concerned. Anyway, gay sex was considered dirty, unnatural and to be condemned. What more: gays did not seek lasting, monogamous relationships. Conversely, heterosexuals

67

had the secure haven of matrimony, which automatically protected them from HIV or other venereal diseases.

By now, we should know that this is a false conclusion. The haven of matrimony has both an entrance as well as an exit. There are plenty of men who cheat on their wives and vice versa. Furthermore, in Germany the number of marriages has decreased for many years, while the number of divorces has been increasing. In major cities, the number of single households is growing steadily. There is enough opportunity for extramarital activity. And that certainly is not only in Germany.

German statistics show that six condoms are used per man per year based on the whole male population from babies to senior citizens. Narrowed to the sexually active population, it might be twelve condoms per year. Even the 16th century was more open and less uptight. Believe it or not, MARTIN LUTHER (1483 – 1546), the renowned German reformer and founder of the Protestant church, can be quoted for sexual advice: »*Twice a week does no harm to him or her.*« If Luther's quote still holds true, the average heterosexual couple has intercourse about a hundred times per year, and mostly unprotected. Conversely, the majority of German homosexuals is opting for safe sex. And that certainly does not only apply to Germany, either.

Nevertheless, a condom can add joy and commonality to a satisfying sex life. Once a heterosexual colleague asked me, if I used condoms. »*Yes*«, I nodded. »*Black ones.*«

»*But you can't see them!*«, he replied obviously confused.

Me: »*Seems like heterosexuals have less imagination!*«

IT HAS NOTHING TO DO WITH ME

It happens in the best families: a marriage ends in divorce, and the following relationship does not work out either. What does the experienced man or woman do when tired of being alone? The same as everyone else does. Before dating online, people went to bars and discotheques to find someone for a night or more. Today it is the chat room or the dating portal that creates the hook up. Is HIV a topic when it comes to one-night-stands? »*Nope*«, you regularly and illogically hear, »*that's something to deal with when the relationship becomes more serious*.« So unprotected intercourse seems to be normal among heterosexuals and outnumbers any gay habits by far. So much for gay men being a high-risk group. And why should heterosexuals not be threatened by venereal diseases including HIV?

It is not only the physical threat of a sickness that gets to people, but more the fear. It is the fear of being unattractive due to the virus, the fear of facing a life of being single – without children and grandchildren, and the fear of being a misfit. Beyond that, it is the fear of suddenly being confronted by and involved with something that has up to then been associated with others. No longer: HIV is not only the sickness of the others. It can happen to anyone, to people who lead so-called normal lives, who mow the lawn, sweep the sidewalk, take out the trash, wash their car, are proud of their preppy kids and lead an outwardly life above reproach. These are people who think they are safe because they deflect the risk for HIV onto gays and drug addicts. But unprotected casual sex can lead to infections with STDs including HIV. So they should think about the consequences, before they have a night of too much booze and a one-night-stand, before they visit a brothel or have a quickie at the party. Suddenly, they are forced to deal with an unknown danger. Having cheated on their spouses, they fear having been infected with anything; and anything in most cases means HIV, because that would be the ultimate punishment. It is not the threat itself, but rather the guilty conscience that makes them quake. And believe it or not, they are consulting the worldwide web instead of seeing a doctor.

I have been working for an HIV online forum for more than six years now. Again and again, I encounter the same situations, questions and fear of the consequences. The

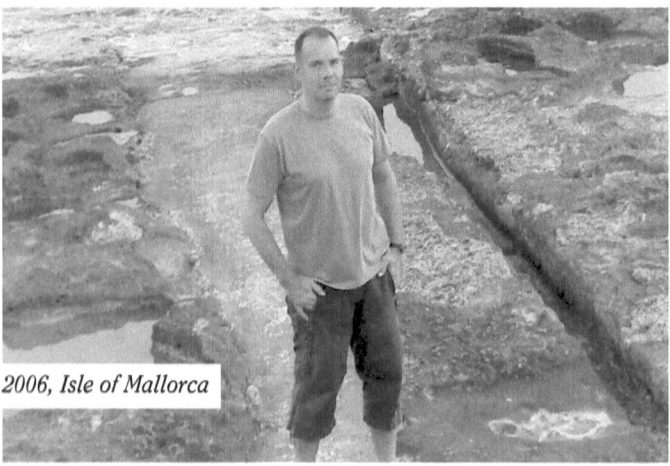

2006, Isle of Mallorca

users fear having contracted *it,* fear being unmasked as a cheater by their partner, neighbor or colleague, or even worse, fear of being found out as gay or bisexual. The users want to cut to the chase as quickly as possible, get to the heart of the matter, but an HIV test takes time to be conclusive. These weeks of waiting are the worst time imaginable. It is not only the risk of an infection, but the number of excuses that need to be invented for not having sex with one's partner. The excuses run out quickly. And what is the next step? Instead of being honest, many people try to distract from their guilt. It is not uncommon that they pretend indignation that others lack faith in them.

But the virus does not care if its host is male or female, hetero-, bi- or homosexual. Unless heterosexuals specifically do not accept this fact, there will be questions like: »*Can I get the infection by kissing someone?*«, »*Can I get the infection by sharing a cigarette with a HIV positive person?*«, »*Can I get the infection by touching a blood stain on a cardboard box?*« or »*Can I get the infection using the same glass as an HIV positive person?*« And the answer will always be: »*No, you can't.*« But every time I get questions like that, my memory goes back to magazines of the 70s, when female teenagers asked anxiously if they could have gotten pregnant by kissing their boyfriends.

The ignorance of anything related to HIV still leads to various forms of discrimination. HIV infected women are stereotyped as leading an amoral life; heterosexual HIV positive men are supposed to be gay; and gay men as a whole are suspected of being infected anyway.

In 2009/2010, a court case received a lot of media attention in Germany. The singer of a nation-wide renowned girl band was accused of having infected her former lover with HIV some five years earlier. During the trial, she admitted to have kept her infection secret for years out of fear of not finding a partner. Her ex-lover certainly had led a life full of pleasure since then and even boasted in court that he, out of principle, only had unprotected intercourse. According to German law the singer was sentenced to two years and released on probation.

During this court case, a heterosexual HIV positive friend and I posted a statement in the online forum of Germany's biggest women magazine. The statement dealt with the *principle of a shared responsibility* with HIV, and had been published shortly before that by the German AIDS self-help organization. The statement concluded that both partners having sexual intercourse are urged to be responsible for their own protection. Although that sounds reasonable, the ladies (and few men) in the online forum did not accept that. On one hand, they declared that discrimination of HIV infected people no longer existed. Conversely, they unanimously agreed that an HIV positive person always had to disclose his or her status, whether in treatment or not. That judgment actually leads to false security: if disclosure of HIV is obligatory, does a non-disclosure mean that there is no HIV? Even in developed countries many people carry the virus without knowing it. They are the ones who continue to spread the infection. In Germany there are an estimated 15,000 people who do not know about their HIV infection.

Very soon the tone of the discussion changed. Although the case affected a woman, suddenly, homosexuals became the main topic. One female user commented: »*There is no civil right for indiscriminate screwing around, even if gay people don't like to hear that.*« And shortly after that, she added rape, pedophilia and HIV to be one and the same thing. Others were not as impertinent and illogical. But they stuck to their belief that honesty about the HIV status was essential when it comes to sexual encounters. Only that way the negative partner can decide how to cope with the situation. Of course, this was only an excuse. To emphasize this, I outlined a situation and asked the users to describe their reaction: »*Two people of any sex meet in a bar. After having flirted for some time, they mutually decide to go to bed. One of the two is you. Suddenly the other person reveals he/she is HIV positive. As I have understood so far, a sexual encounter with a positive person is completely out of question. How do you explain your sudden change of mind and manage to get out of this situation?*«

There were no less than three [!] answers, but they all dealt more with the situation than with the question.

Answer one: »*I am furious.*«

Why furious? Are we talking about the honesty that some postings ago had unequivocally been demanded? Or are we talking about the wasted time and energy for flirting?

Answer two: »*I would leave immediately, without a word.*«

If that happened to you, wouldn't you think twice about being honest the next time?

Answer three: »*I feel nauseous.*«

That is the only more or less honest answer out of the three, because it still leaves the opportunity to talk. The other two answers are nothing but discrimination and are only based on the false assumption that HIV only affects the others. But this is, and remains, prejudice. And it can be overcome only with knowledge and information, because it is quite simply a question of health. And health is too precious to let others decide for you. So those who protect themselves, share the responsibility.

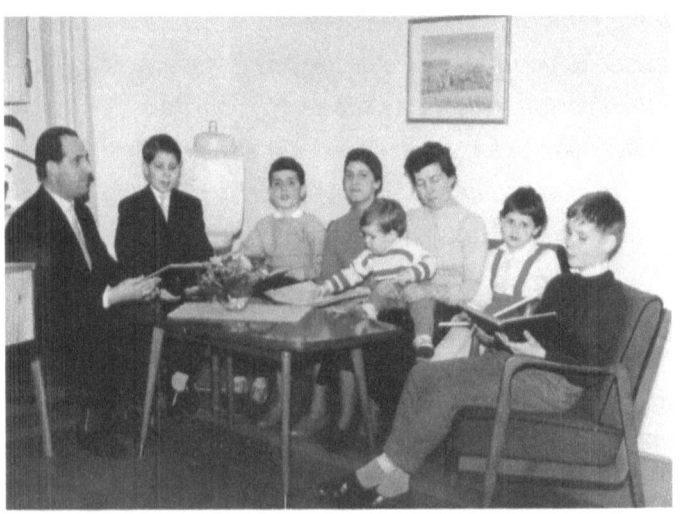

1960: Sunday afternoon at the Gerschwitz' living-room.
All are singing, except for the one on mom's lap: me.

LUST FOR LIFE

You do not change your whole life just because of some virus wreaks havoc in your blood. Well, you get anxious about a cold, pimples or a sudden pain, and wonder if it is due to the infection. Additionally, lots of buzzwords are circulating that fuel insecurity and fear: opportunistic infections, the collapse of the immune system or the final outbreak of AIDS. No one talks about opportunistic infections unless the immune system is weakened, and only then, do they come into limelight. Diseases like pneumonia or toxoplasmosis, provoked by viruses, bacteria, parasites or fungi, do not harm healthy people, but they can be life threatening for those with a weak immune system. An opportunistic infection is the first sign of the immune system breaking down, thus marking the transition from a positive HIV status to AIDS. In 1994, when I received the diagnosis, this development was a foregone conclusion. Predicting I would lead a relatively healthy and symptom-free life more than twenty years after the initial diagnosis would have been called pure fantasy and a rejection of reality. Even thinking of that was absurd in those days. Thank God this has changed for the better. Opportunistic infections are still a threat, but with antiretroviral treatment stabilizing the immune system, they do not occur that often any more. Accordingly, life expectancy has risen significantly. Today thanks to the medication, even HIV positive people are expected to live as long as negative people.

In the early days of 1994, when I had not yet internalized my infection, I made a big mistake. As I carefully sought to enlarge my rather rudimentary knowledge of HIV, I went to the movies with a friend to see »*And the Band Played On*«. Based on true events, the 1993 movie tells the story of HIV and AIDS from the very beginning in the early 80s. It describes the helplessness of doctors, the scientists' race for a cure and the suffering of those infected, whose future showed nothing other than death. It was a very realistic portrayal, but it came way too early for me. I was not really able to deal with the topic only a few months after my diagnosis. I had no guidance and was more or less alone in unchartered territory.

What did I learn from that?

Nothing.

A couple of months later I went to see »*Philadelphia*«, the first commercial Hollywood movie dealing with AIDS. In the meantime, I had become a bit more familiar with the disease, but was still mentally stressed. This time, it was not the confrontation with the inevitability of death, but the outlook how it might happen. I refused to think of an end as miserable as shown in Tom Hanks' performance. Remember: he acted so well that he was awarded an Oscar©.

By the way: »*Philadelphia*« is a perfect example for selective perception. The disease is only part of the subplot; the main storyline deals with the discrimination against the AIDS patient by his employer and his ensuing efforts for rehabilitation. This part of the plot turns out to be successful because the protagonist wins at the end. But the message that stayed with me did not have a happy-end: Andrew Beckett (Tom Hanks) dies. And that made it clear again: HIV is incurable; the infection inevitably leads to death.

It took another twelve to eighteen months until I finally accepted and internalized the infection. These were months full of insecurity. I neither had the slightest clue about the effects of the infection on my professional and social life, nor did I know anything about how my health would develop. On the other hand, it was a time for action. I tried to answer every question mark regarding the future with an exclamation mark full of optimism. And I distracted myself by working hard and going out to bars. Looking back, 1994 and 1995 actually turned out to be the most exciting years of self-employment even though I was emotionally confused. The spectrum of my work included organizational tasks as well as the development of marketing and product concepts for fragrances and body care products. Furthermore, I met a lot of new people, many of whom are still good friends today. That was soothing to the soul. Many small, but beautiful, moments strengthened my self-confidence, and professional success attested to the unbroken creativity and drive.

Nevertheless, I still did not talk about HIV, although it was submerged and churned in me. Even the best distraction could not conceal the fact I myself had not yet come to terms with my incomprehensible disease. Sometimes I wanted to bluster, loose my cool, get upset and just talk, at other times I was still afraid to do so.

Friends I took into my confidence were just as helpless. When someone suggested that I should seek professional support I categorically refused. Not that I did not trust in psychology or psychologists, but I was used to handling problems on my own. As the youngest of six siblings, I had learned to come out on top, most likely due to the bonus of being the pet of the family. My brothers and sisters all went into the music business with violin, cello, viola or keyboards. I instead ventured onto a new path: I studied marketing and advertising. My dad probably would have liked me to also follow the musical family tradition, but my mom was quite happy that she had another topic of conversation from at least one of the kids.

Sometimes my attempts to resolve the situation on my own were interpreted as weakness. »*You don't want to be helped*«, I often heard. On the outside, it probably looked like I could not (or would not) open up to others. The reason was completely different: I was afraid to be confronted with too much knowledge about HIV and AIDS. Until then, I had collected information only selectively. It could have easily been more, but sometimes too many facts have the connotation of something final, unchangeable, irreversible. The state of knowledge 1994/ 1995 did not bode well. Remembering the negative experience with the two movies, I was not willing to expose myself to that again. So I decided to choose another way to deal with it.

If you are not exactly in the know about something, you

are allowed to cherish even the most irrational hopes. I did hope to control the disease progress by pure optimism. I was not going to let that dumb virus get the better of me! By coincidence, I found a quotation by a German writer that proved my idea right: »*He, who can laugh when he should have sobbed will find back to the joy of living.*« I entered the fray: virus versus imperturbable optimism. Although it sounded like an unequal battle, I finally had vanquished insecurity.

Now that I had accepted the infection as something normal, I started to look at it from different perspectives. It had taken me about eighteen months to cope with the life-changing diagnosis. Actually, that was quite fast. Although I had been shocked, I was not shaken to the core. In the last years, I have witnessed some different ways to cope: people younger than me fled into sex, drugs and rock 'n' roll because they had lost future alternatives. Persons my age bemoaned their fate and became cold, mean and cynical, even to hitherto good friends, because they had to fight both the encroaching midlife crisis and the infection.

Looking back I have learned one thing: even when you are HIV positive, life goes on. Although the first months were dominated by fears, insecurity and lethargy, I soon found out that these emotions were not dictated externally, but internally. And therefore I was able to exert influence on them. If you use the positive psychosomatic opportunities, – even the Bible knows »*A cheerful heart is good medicine*« (Proverbs 17,22) – so the soul can add a lot to strengthen the immune system. Nevertheless, even the greatest optimism cannot guarantee keeping the virus in check. The day inevitably comes when treatment is necessary. That is the day of the biggest change in life. Now you can see the infection in terms of medication piling up in your kitchen, bathroom or bedroom. Medication you have to take from now on until the end of your life. Although there has been a huge progress in research and development, the effectiveness of treatment has been significantly improved and the side effects have been reduced, treatment will not work without pills, and it affects daily life. Taking medicine has to become a routine, once or twice a day. They still are a kind of a foreign body, even if it is clear that they are the only warranty for a life as long and healthy as possible.

In meanwhile fifteen years of treatment, I have not always succeeded in sticking to my pill regimen. So sometimes I just forgot, sometimes I denied it. Once I even thought I could outfox the virus by the strong belief in some kind of the self-healing power of positive thinking. Since I felt healthy and strong, I decided I no longer needed medication and interrupted treatment without consulting my doctor. Actually, I wanted to be free of the side effects, even though I had known from the beginning they occurred. I stopped taking the pills.

When the doctor checked my blood again about a year later, I told him. He was simply furious: »*In my practice all HIV patients are under the virus detection limit. I won't let you mess up with these outstanding results. You are not going to ruin my statistics!*«

Most likely I needed such a clear, emphatic reminder. I felt healthy, but my blood values proved the opposite. So I had no choice but to accept the necessity of taking my pills regularly. That became even clearer, when I received a second kick in the ass: I contracted pneumonia caused by legionella. Although this is not listed as an opportunistic infection, the experience proved its point. Compliance, taking your medication exactly as prescribed, is essential.

Since then, I have preferred to live with the side effects. I suffer from insomnia and the consequential fatigue during the day. I need more time in the morning to get going and I need to rest around noon. Luckily, I am self-employed and work at home, so I can integrate all this into my daily routine without problems. As long as these are the only side effects, I sure can live with them.

After more than twenty years HIV has become normality to me. If I had not written books about it, I probably would not think about the infection as much. But I received so many positive reactions on the books from both HIV negative and positive people that I am certain I did the right thing. As I am open about HIV, work for a newsgroup and lecture on HIV and prevention, an increasing number of people, not only friends and acquaintances, ask me for advice, particularly when there is a recent diagnosis. I fully understand the anxieties and insecurities that such a blow causes. It may not help in the very first moment, but there is a reliable truth: HIV today is not a death sentence and one's quality of life is not dramatically affected anymore.

Take me as an example. With a viral load below the detection limit, my immune system works as well as if there was no HIV. Since I have known about my diagnosis, I have started to live more consciously and to enjoy life, maybe even more than before. I pruned my address book of false friends and kept the good ones. I found out about friendship: it is too rare and too precious to flog dead horses.

YOLO – you only live once.
You see: I did not lose my sense of humor to the virus.

My feet are firmly planted on the ground; my thoughts circle around my existence much more intensively than before. Thanks to my optimism, I do not worry about the future. The necessity of accepting a diagnosis like HIV offered me the chance of inventing a new sight to life and set me on the right track to a positive future – and I mean exactly that: positive in every way. Of course, this is neither a testimony in favor of the infection nor a trivialization of it. On the contrary: I wish everybody to stay HIV negative forever. But even being HIV positive, you can enjoy life. This is actually what this book is all about: no more and no less.

Because there is a life beyond the virus.

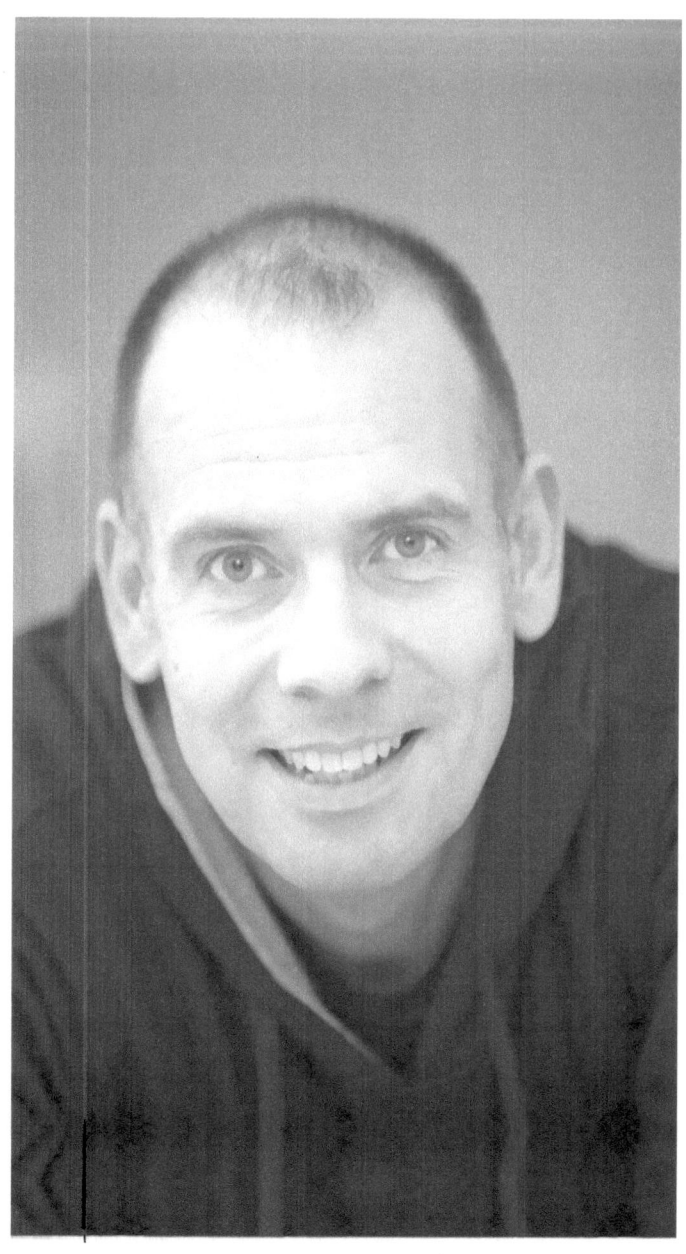